ABSESSION

www.fitforfaithministries.com

America's Guide to Ultimate **6** Pack Abs

Author By

SCOTT HAYWARD, CPT, CSCS

AB SESSION

Table of Contents

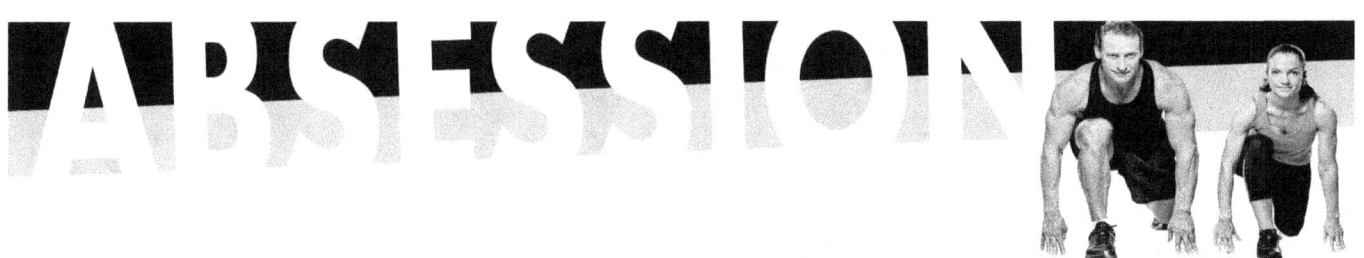

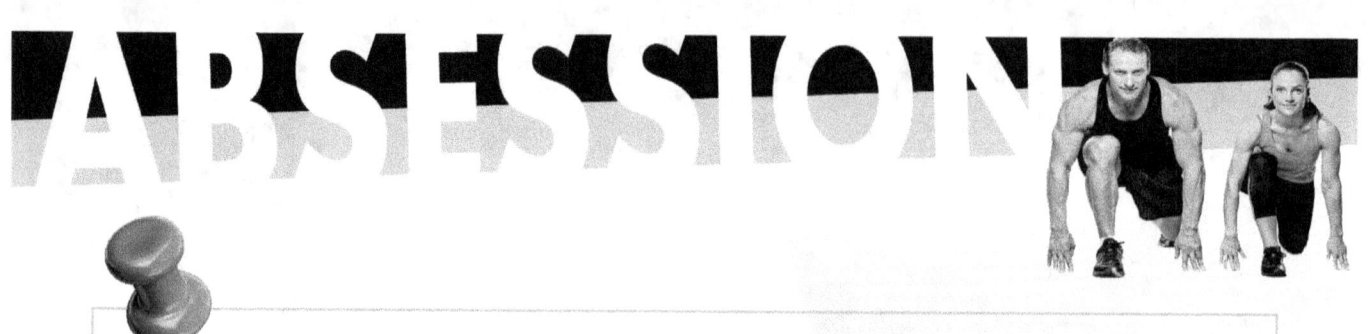

NOTICE of LIABILITY

There are inherent risks with all forms of exercise. Readers are advised to take full responsibility for their safety and the safety of others they are training.

Before beginning any exercise, be sure the equipment you will be using is in proper working order.

Know your limits and do not take risks beyond your level of experience in training and fitness. The exercise and diet information contained in the book is not meant to substitute any treatment or diet that may have been prescribed by a doctor.

As with all exercise programs and diets, obtain a doctor's approval before beginning. While every precaution has been taken in the preparation of this book, the author shall have no liability to any persons or entity with respect to loss, damage or injury caused or alleged to be caused directly or indirectly by the instructions contained in this book or the exercise instructions contained herein

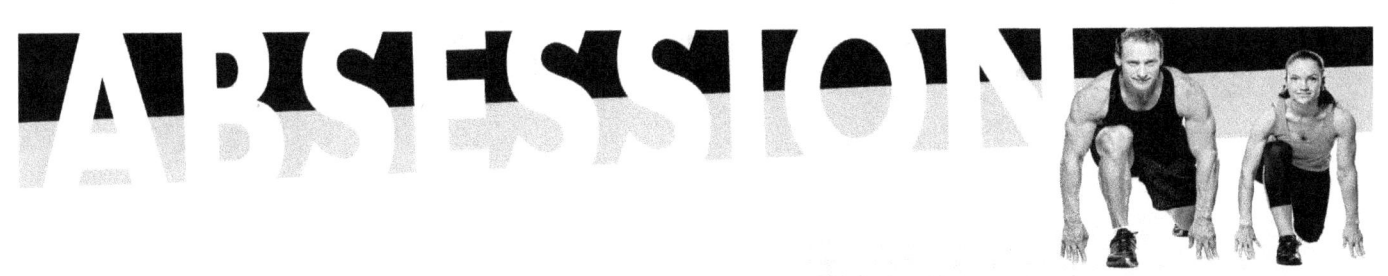

AB SESSION

Dedicated to those of you that takes this opportunity
to change your body and
ultimately change your life —forever!

ABSESSION

A book of this type (or any type) is hardly ever a work of just one person. So, as I started to thinkof all the people that I wanted to thank for making this book a reality, the list grew on and on.

First of all, I thank my Lord and Savior Jesus Christ. Whom without his guidance and everlasting support I am nothing. Next, I would like to thank my daughters Jordan and McKenna. They are the driving force behind me. Their lives constantly challenge and encourage me to become more than I was the day before. I owe a debt of gratitude to my mother, who has always believed in and supported me wholeheartedly.

Then, there were the sympathetic ears of Jason Wilson and Tracy Wagner. They both encouraged and endured my ramblings and re-ramblings as I composed this body of work.

I would also like to thank my technical go-to guys Thomas Rueli and Joseph Vuotto who put up with change after change with regards to the set-up and proofing of this book.

And last but not least, I would like to thank Mr. Brian McCall, who challenged me to strive to achieve more given a bad a set of circumstances and to take heart the truths presented in Romans 8:28.

I would also like to thank YOU for taking the opportunity to read this book and ultimately change your life.

To all of these people and countless others that have stood by me and helped shape the person I have become - Thank You.

I was extremely honored when Scott asked me to write the forward for his new book. I've known Scott for over 6 years and I always thought he should write a book, to dispel some of the fitness folk lore and myths that have pervaded late night infomercials and society as a whole.

I have been training for over 20 years and have competed on the amateur and professional levels. In all my time involved in fitness, I have never met a more knowledgeable, innovative and forward thinking trainer and fitness professional than Scott Hayward. He takes the most difficult concepts of exercise physiology and exercise kinesiology and puts them in everyday-language so you and I can see how to apply it to our lives.

In all of my time involved in the fitness industry, I have seen many books written about nutrition, workouts and especially training abs. This book is by far the best read that doesn't miss anything. I know this book is based around achieving a better set of Abdominals, but in reality, Scott has given you the recipe for success not only for achieving a better body, but a better, more fulfilling life.

This book can benefit anyone looking to get the most out of their body and ultimately their life. I've thoroughly enjoyed reading this book and can't wait to implement some of his training and nutrition advice into my next contest prep.

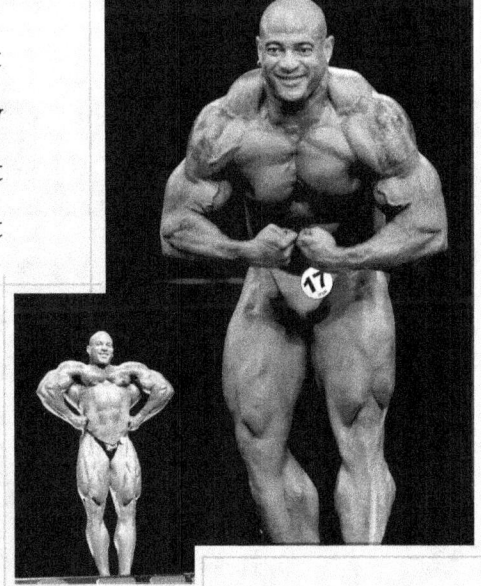

Great job on this book, I can't wait to read the next one.

Fauzi Hanst
IFBB Pro Bodybuilder

ABSESSION

While putting together my notes for this book, I've talked to thousands of people. When asked the question; "What body part do you wish you could improve?" Answers were almost unanimous - ABS!! The funny thing is I spoke to people from all walks of life and abdominal muscles. Whether you call Rectus Abdominis, Abs, 6 pack or (for the few genetically gifted), 8 pack, everybody wants a toner, leaner, more streamlined mid-section.

America is obsessed (or more aptly put) absessed with their waistlines. It's flaunted every-where you look. Television, billboards, print ads, movies, music videos - all throughout the media, a set of well defined Abdominals are celebrated and much coveted.

The one common problem I had discovered interviewing these people was no one answer existed to the question; "How do I get a six pack?" Replies were as varied as the size of the people to whom I spoke. Hi-protein, no carbs, drink water, drink no water, wear a garbage bag while running (I liked that one a lot), do lots of cardio, do no cardio, do 5,000 crunches a day (a close runner up for my favorite), the list goes on and on. Each answer proved my point. No one commanded the TRUTH, the key to obtaining a set of washboard abdominals. One poor misguided soul who was wearing $29.95 around his waist (the rubber and Velcro belt) said; "Eat garlic, it takes the fat from the inside out." This guy actually had two rubber type belts sewn together to make it around his girth!

With all of this misinformation, I decided to write a definitive book on the What's, Where's, When's, and Why's of developing a lean, defined, chiseled mid-section. This manual will cover all the disciplines required to develope your very own coveted prize. We will discuss Aerobic and Anaerobic Exercise, Nutrition, Energy Systems, Resistance Training and Specific Abdominal Exercises, all specifically tailored to fit within a convenient fitness regiment.

Obtaining a 6 pack is not the destination, but rather the journey. Not only will you become leaner, but you will be engaged in a complete body makeover, developing sculpted shoulders, a chiseled chest, a broadened back and an enhanced V-Taper. Aside from the aesthetics, you will also reduce your chance of coronary disease and stress, promoted better sex, overall lead a more productive, fulfilling life and possibly add years to your life.

If you are pessimistic concerning your individual potential for success of improving your physique and ultimately your life, don't be. Read on –Other than your spare tire, what do you have to lose?

Any book, exercise gizmo, or program that doesn't encompass a holistic approach to developing a 6 pack isn't going to be successful. The only way to ensure that you will meet your desired outcome is through a comprehensive all-inclusive plan. With the goal of a six pack firmly implanted, the approach must include all of the following: Resistance Training, Cardiovascular/ Aerobic Training and a Sound Nutritional Program. Without one of these components, you are setting yourself up for failure.

You're A.B.S. Holistic Approach to achieving your six pack will look like this:

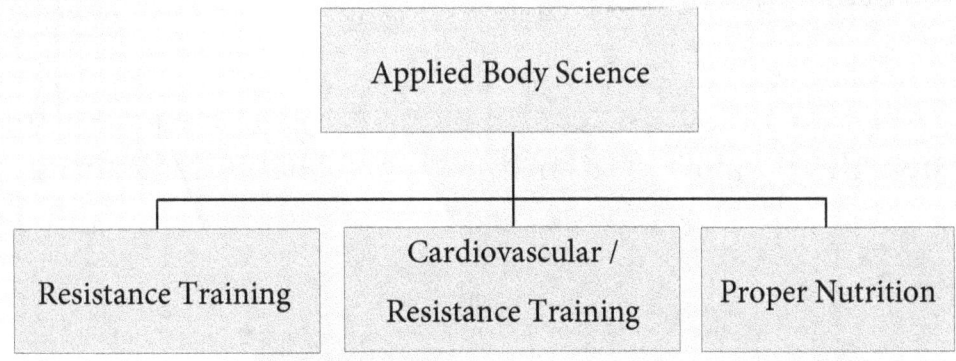

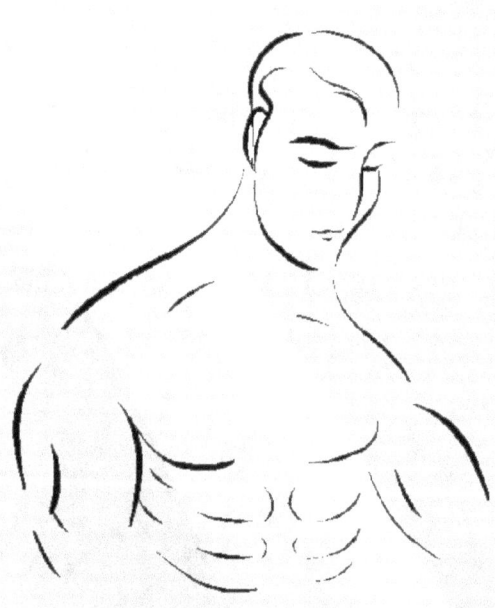

The person who makes a success of living is the one who sees his goal steadily and aims for it unswervingly. That is dedication.

- Cecil B. DeMille

ABSESSION

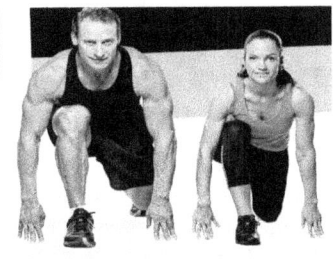

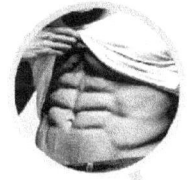

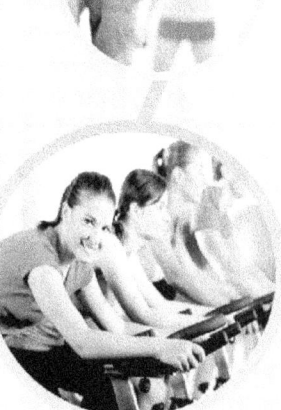

Before you jump into your sweatsuit and start crunching away like a wide-eyed maniac, let's discuss biological energy systems for a moment. These systems are simple to understand; they are where your body gets its energy and are as important as the exercise you perform for fat loss. So if you can understand how you body works then you'll better appreciate how to train your body in order to achieve the results you desire.

Energy Systems are an often overlooked, but critical piece to the puzzle in achieving your best body. Each of us requires a currency of energy for life. The source of which is a molecule called Adenosine Tri-Phosphate or ATP for short. The body uses ATP for all of its energy needs and consequently for all biological functions. Without ATP muscles can neither contract nor relax. Actually without ATP you will die—rigor mortis sets in. Let's take a closer look at how this incredibly important ATP is manufactured.

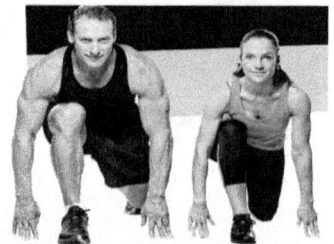

ATP – CP SYSTEM

The first of the three Energy Systems we will look at is the ATP-CP System. The energy molecule ATP is readily manufactured in tiny structures called mitochondria (the power house) inside each human. ATP is nothing more than one Adenosine molecule connected (or bonded) to three phosphates. When one of the phosphates disengages or is released from ATP energy is released. This energy then becomes readily available in the muscles for quick bursts of energy. When a phosphate is disassociated from ATP, another critical molecule Creatine Phosphate (CP) lends one of its phosphates to resynthesize the original by-product Adenosine Di-Phosphate (ADP) back into ATP. This energy system is usually the major contributor for the first 30 seconds of a high intensity activity. A capsulated answer to why you need to rest in between sets of heavy resistance training assuming you want to reach the same, or close to the same number of repetitions set to set. I know it is a little confusing so here is a diagram to make it a little easier to comprehend.

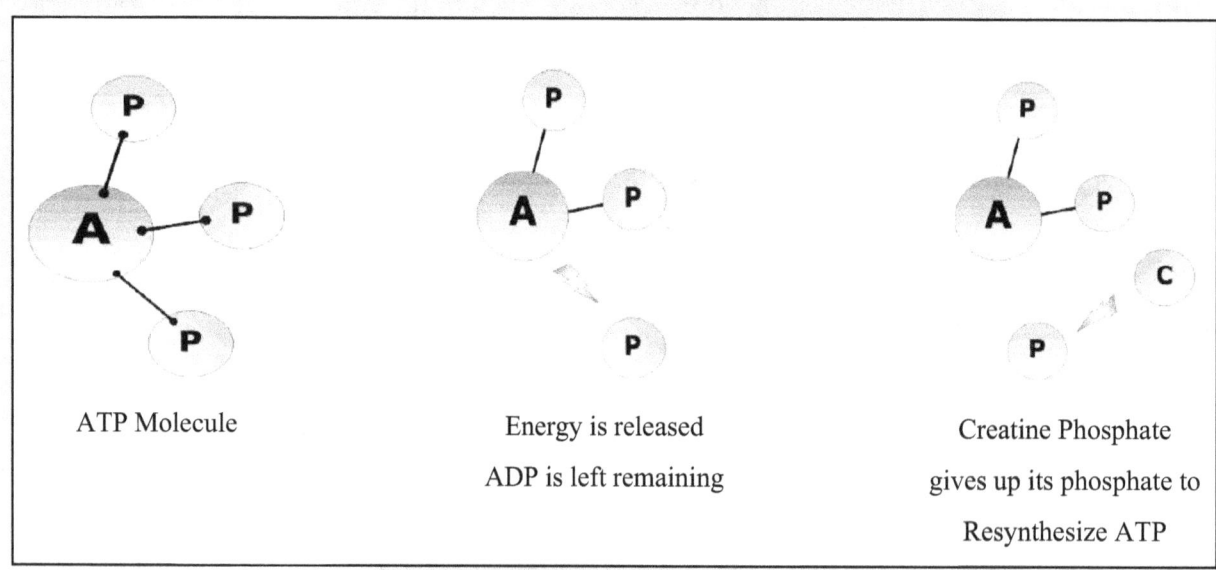

ATP Molecule

Energy is released
ADP is left remaining

Creatine Phosphate
gives up its phosphate to
Resynthesize ATP

On the surface this ostensibly appears to be a great way to do business, to release energy from an energy containing molecule and regenerate it. Case closed. Not so fast my friend! The AT-PCP system only lasts for approximately 30 seconds, enough for short bursts. But what happens then? Read on, Read on ….

Let me start off by saying, all energy systems are constantly working, but at different percentages based on energy demand (intensity) and the length of duration needed for that demand. Energy production is neither compartmentalized nor linear, when one energy system shuts down another may or may not pick up where the former left off. Our bodies are so much more efficient than that.

The second energy system we will discuss is what is called Anaerobic Glycolysis. Well, translating the name we can pretty much break down what is going on. Anaerobic means "without the presence of oxygen", and Glycolysis (hold on to your heads), Glyco means "sugar" and lysis translates "to break apart." So together we have the breaking apart of sugar without oxygen. For any of you that remember your 10th grade chemistry class, this next part will be a trip down memory lane.

$C6H12O6$ is the chemical symbol for sugar. That simply means there are 6 Carbon, 12 Hydrogen, and 6 Oxygen molecules; together they comprise one molecule of sugar. In order to break down this structure into a useable energy source the body breaks the 6 Carbon chain into 2 3 Carbon chains the resultant molecule is called pyruvate.

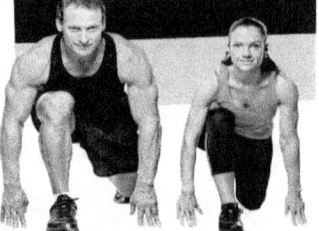

$$C_6 \ H_{12} \ O_6$$

[PYRUVATE]

$$C = C = C \qquad C = C = C$$

From here, the body senses the presence or absence of oxygen. If not enough oxygen exists, a rise of Lactate Acid will occur in the bloodstream. The body will start to shuttle this lactic acid to the liver for storage through a process called the Cory Cycle where it is subsequently stored as an energy source at a later time. At this point your body either slows down to renew oxygen or the muscle becomes so acidic it shuts down. If the intensity continues unabated, the polarity of the muscle changes, which is the acidic value, rises to a point when the muscle must stop or slow down.

If there is sufficient available oxygen, 2 out of the 3 Carbons are converted into Acetyl CoA. Which I like to refer to as the Gatekeeper. Just for the record, the 3rd Carbon is exhaled as Carbon Dioxide. The logic involved with the term gatekeeper is based on the role Acetyl Co enzyme A plays as the "control valve" into the Krebs Cycle.

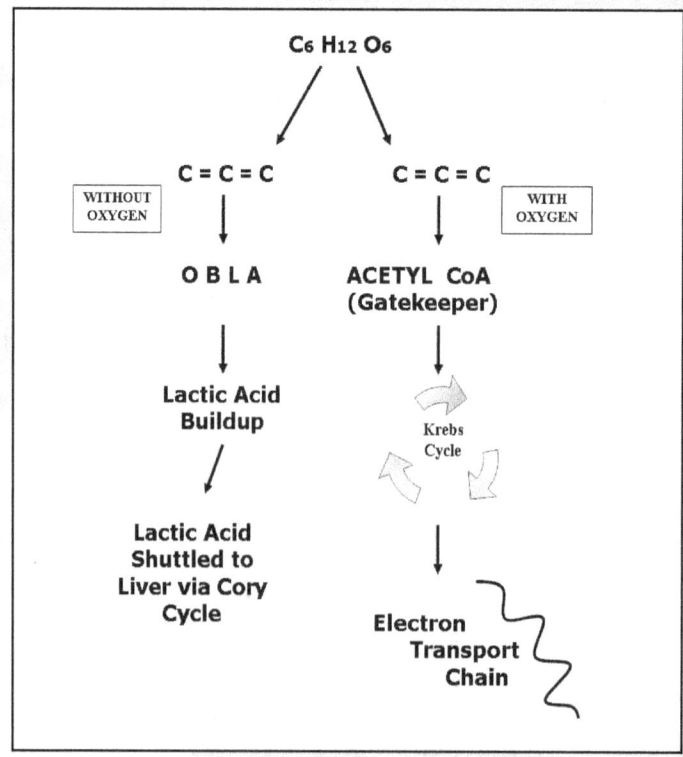

KREBS CYCLE

The easiest way to explain the role of the Krebs Cycle is to envision a Ferris wheel miniaturized down to Cellular Level. As the Carbons are spun around the Ferris wheel and ATPs and electrons are spun off at the rate of 3 ATP's and 3 electrons per cycle. The ATPs are used for energy and the electrons head down the electron transport chain, where they are incorporated into other biological processes.

The most important thing to remember is one molecule of sugar, $C6 - H12 - O6$ produces 38 molecules of ATP. The ongoing metabolic processes involved utilize 2 ATP molecules, leaving you with a net gain of 36 ATPs. This energy system is kick started predominantly in the 1 – 3 minute range.

BETA OXIDATION

The third energy system we will discuss is Beta-Oxidation. If you want to lose fat, **READ THIS SECTION CAREFULLY.**

A Fat molecule is comprised of one glycerol molecule and three molecules of varying fatty acids (See Figure 1). A Triglyceride is the body's molecule storage for excess calories. Your body has a built in survival mechanism that is constantly storing any overabundance of calories like that extra slice of pizza consumed, mindlessly preparing for an impending famine (lucky you.)

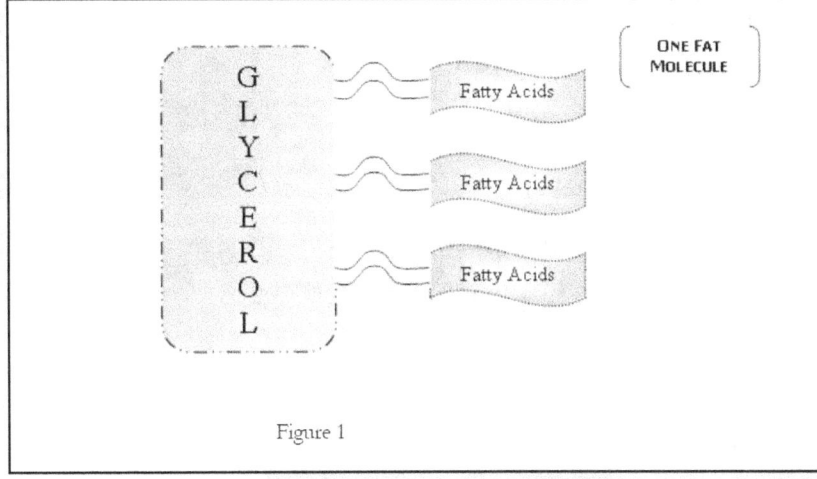

Figure 1

In order to use this stored energy, chemical bonds must be broken down. Initially, the bonds between the glycerol and the fatty acids are hydrolyzed. Water breaks apart those bonds (See Figure 2). Then, the fatty acids are oxidized- this oxidation breaks the fatty acids into nine pairs of carbons per fatty acid.

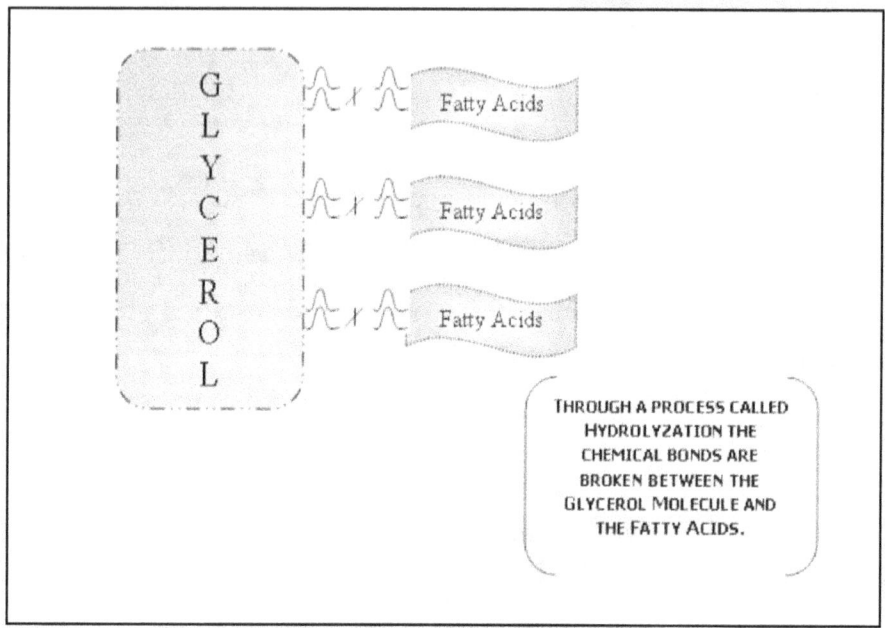

THROUGH A PROCESS CALLED HYDROLYZATION THE CHEMICAL BONDS ARE BROKEN BETWEEN THE GLYCEROL MOLECULE AND THE FATTY ACIDS.

Now that you have generated carbon pairs, they can be converted into Acetyl CoA, The Gatekeeper. Then funneled back into the Krebs Cycle- spitting out ATP's and electrons.

Once, ATP is kicked out of the Krebs Cycle, it is employed as an energy source and the electrons are sent down the electron transport chain (ETC). Simply put, think of a set of stairs. At the top rests a metal slinky, that toy you played with as a child. As the slinky (the electron), descends the stairs, it kicks out an ATP with each step.

Remember, all 3 systems are always working, just in different proportions.

The percentage of participation by all 3 energy systems is determined by the duration of the exercise and the intensity of the exercise.

Some quick notes on the Beta-Oxidation Energy System: the fat molecule must first be hydro-lyzed the process begins with hydrolyzed triglycerides promoted in the presence of oxygen, supplied in the form of water. That's why plenty of water is crucial. So, in summary 460 ATPs are produced per 1 triglyceride- there are some conditions that need to be met:

- Sufficient Oxygen
- Plenty of Water
- Sufficient Time > 16 – 20 minutes

Well, that is our trip through chemistry and discovering "how" your body makes and uses ATP.

Energy Systtem	ATP/CP Systtem	Anaerobiic Gllycollysiis	Betta Oxiidattiion
Functions Aerobically or Anaerobically	Anaerobic in nature	Anaerobic in nature	Anaerobic in nature
Energy used for:	Immediate	Short Term	Long Term
Uses for Energy	Stored ATP/CP in muscles	Glycogen	Fatty Acids
Endurance	Fatigues easily	Moderate Fatigue Factor	Longest to Fatigue
Predominant Intensity	High Intensity	High to Moderate Intensity	Moderate to Low intensity
Energy Stores Avail-ability	ATP CP Stores in muscle	36 ATP from one molecule of Sugar	460 ATP from one Triglyceride

The contributing percentage of all 3 energy systems is determined by the duration and the intensity of the activity. The 3 systems are not compartmentalized, starting and stopping before another system kicks in, but rather function simultaneously and seamlessly among each system. This is what is meant when I stated earlier that energy production is neither compartmentalized nor linear, they work together.

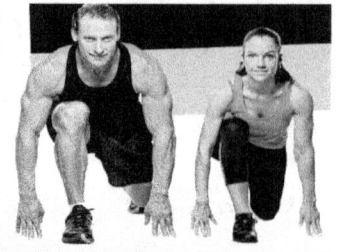

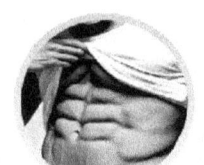

Aerobic Exercise is an activity based on a continuous rhythmic movement for a set period of time, in the presence of oxygen.

Let's breakdown this word "cardiovascular" so it can be more easily understood - Cardio means "heart" and vascular means the "blood", including veins, vessels and capillaries. Often times you will see the word respiratory placed with cardio -Cardiorespiratory - that translates into heart and lungs.

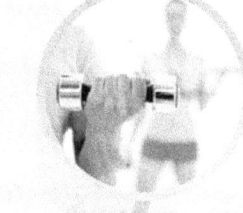

With our fundamental knowledge of energy systems, let's look at ways we might combine this knowledge with cardiovascular exercise to obtain our lean, trim waistline.

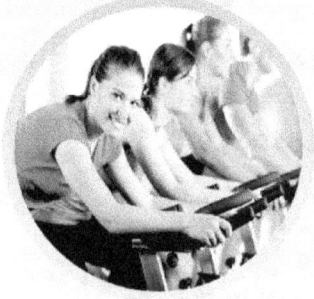

Aerobic activity is a good tool in fighting the battle of the bulge. In addition to burning a large number of calories in a relatively short time, it also ramps up your metabolism after the activity is concluded.

You may be thinking fine, but how long, how fast, what kind of cardiovascular exercise do I perform? These questions are very easily answered using the Personal Training Acronym F.I.T.T.

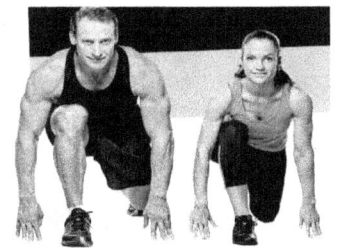

This stands for:

Frequency = How often?

Intensity = How hard?

Time = How long?

Type = What mode of activity?

Don't worry; we will address each of these four components of your cardiovascular prescription in a moment, for now, the most important thing to keep in mind is your ultimate goal-ABS to die for!!!

Since we are examining cardiovascular / aerobic type exercises, this is a good place to look at the most important muscle of all - the heart.

First off, let's go over some of the anatomy before we get to the physiology of the circulatory system. The heart is comprised of 4 chambers – the 2 upper chambers (or atria) and the 2 lower chambers (the ventricles). The hearts starts off with only 2 chambers (one incoming and one outgoing) while in utero, but over time the 2 chambers twist and merge- becoming the 4 chamber heart that we all have.

Blood has two constituent parts, the red blood cells part which contain hemoglobin and the liquid or serum part. Hemoglobin is the oxygen laden molecules transferring oxygen to the other body cells, after dropping off its oxygen it returns to the heart via the superior and inferior vena cava (two large collection veins). The blood then travels to the right atrium, passed through the tricuspid valve to the right ventricle. From the right ventricle, the blood travels to the lungs where it deposits carbon dioxide, picks up oxygen through osmosis, an exchange occurring system by way of thousands of sack-like structures called alveoli. Once the lungs re-oxygenate the blood, it travels to the left atrium, through the bicuspid valve and down into the left ventricle.

(Note: the left ventricle is the thickest of all the quadrants). From the left ventricle, the blood travels out throughout the body via the aorta to the body and working muscles.

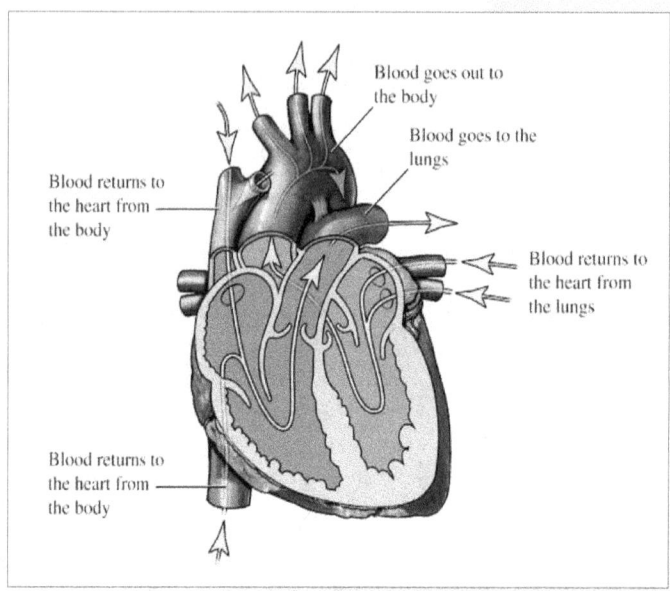

Let's examine some of the chronic affects Cardiovascular Exercise impresses on your body and how. Performing cardiovascular exercise results in physiological changes directly related to overall health improvements and that significantly reduce the risk of coronary heart disease and lung disease. It develops, strengthens and makes the heart, lungs and vascular system more efficient. Your body will specifically change for the better based on the greater demands placed on it during exercise.

Oxygen intake is key here. **VO2 Max**, which is also known as maximal oxygen consumption, is the highest volume of oxygen a person can consume while exercising. This is a person's maximum aerobic capacity. VO2 Max is one of the best measures of maximal cardiovascular performance.

An additional health benefit of cardiovascular training is an increase of cardi-ac output. **Cardiac Output** is the volume of blood expelled by the ventricles of the heat each minute; and is equivalent to the amount of blood ejected at each beat multiplied by the number of beats per minute, usually expressed in liters of blood per minute.

A benefit that goes hand in hand with Cardiac Output is Stroke Volume. Stroke Volume is the amount of blood pumped out per heart beat by the left ventricle. It only makes sense that a correlation exists between these two is, that as Stroke Volume increases, Cardiac Output *must* increase.

Another benefit of cardiovascular training is a marked improvement in Coronary Circulation. Since the heart is a muscle when you exercise a muscle it becomes stronger and bigger (in particular the left ventricular wall) as well as more efficient in all of its functions. Because of this improved circulation and increased blood flow, the diameter of the vessels increase to accommodate the increase activity and blood flow.

In addition to all of these benefits, cardiovascular exercise dramatically affects two very important categories of cardiovascular function. They are; Resting Heart Rate and Blood Pressure. Both are favorably lowered, a true life benefit. If you think about it, it is very easy to un-up, averaged over a three day period. Normally, lower heart rate at rest, is a reliable indicator of aerobic condition. Blood Pressure also improves because it is now easier to move the oxygen and nutrients through the body. Blood pressure is the force exerted against the heart and blood vessel walls by blood in motion. When a blood pressure reading is taken, it is reported as systolic over diastolic value. **Systolic pressure** is caused by the heartbeat or contraction pressure values vary appreciably depending on age, sex, ethnicity and fitness. It is measured with a "cuff" (sphygmomanometer) and measured in, millimeters (mm) of mercury (hg), just like

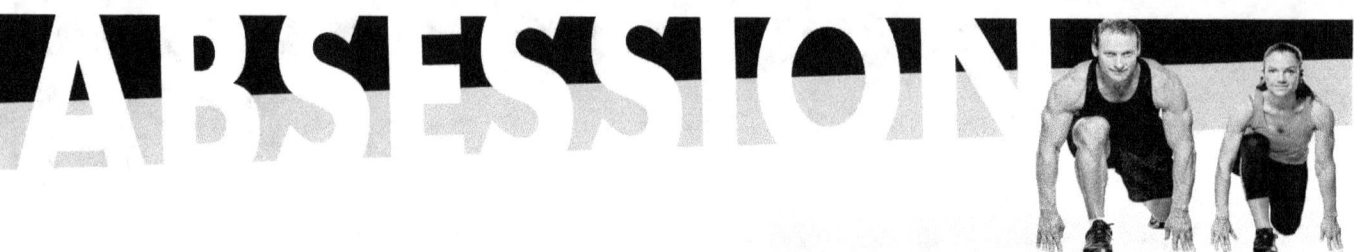

CHRONIC EFFECTS OF CARDIOVASCULAR TRAINING ON THE CARDIOVASCULAR SYSTEM

CHARACTERISTIC	CHANGE
VO2 MAX	⬆
MAXIMAL MET CAPACTIY	⬆
CARDIAC OUTPUT	⬆
STROKE VOLUME	⬆
CORONARY CIRCULATION	⬆
DIAMETER OF VESSELS	⬆
RESTING HEART RATE	⬇
BLOOD PRESSURE	⬇
CARDIAC TISSUE OF LEFT VENTRICULAR WALL	⬆
SIZE OF LEFT VENTRICLE	⬆
CONTRACTILE STATE OF MYOCARDIUM	⬆
PLASMA VOLUME AND TOTAL	⬆
HEMOGLOBIN	⬆
TIDAL VOLUME	⬆

Total =   A HEATHIER BODY

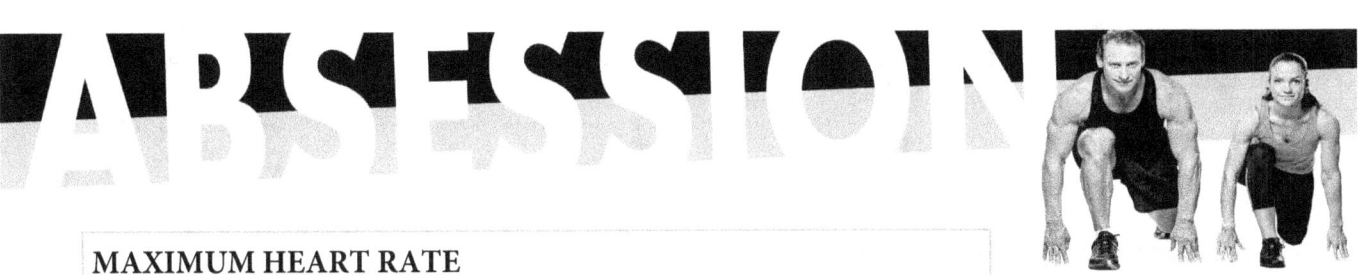

MAXIMUM HEART RATE

To determine exercise intensity we must first determine your maximum heart rate. Simply put, Maximum Heart Rate is the maximal number of times an individual's heart beats within one minute. Maximum heart rate is determined partly by age and partly by genetics. For example, as a newborn your maximal heart is much higher than at 40 or 50 years of age. The clinical method to determine maximal heart rate is employing a Graded Exercise Test administered by a cardiologist or exercise physiologist, but a rough approximation can be obtained with the formula below.

$$220 - Age = Maximum\ Heart\ Rate$$

Now that we have examined coronary circulation and the chronic affects of cardiovascular training on the coronary system, let's examine the components of F.I.T.T., which stands for Frequency, Intensity, Time and Type. Through examining these components, you can determine what kind, how much, how often and how intense you will perform your cardiovascular exercise. By manipulating these variables you can elicit the response you desire from your body.

FREQUENCY

To effectively lose perform 4 -5 cardio sessions a week. These sessions should be split up between two different types of cardio; 1) low intensity steady-state aerobics and 2) higher intensity shorter duration- interval type of training. Both types of cardio have their benefits, and both have their place in the arsenal on fat loss.

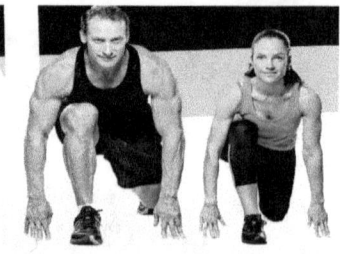

INTENSITY

Low intensity steady state aerobics is best achieved at 60-70% of the maximum heart rate and has been shown to use a predominantly high percentage of fat (triglycerides) as energy. This correlates to a 3 - 4 on the Rate of Perceived Exertion Scale. The Rate of Perceived Exertion is a subjective way to gauge your intensity level during exercise.

Once you have determined your maximal heart rates using the formula above now take your MHR and multiply it by .60 for the lower end and .70 for the upper end to obtain your heart rate bell curve.

This is your target heart rate (THR):

Example 220 – 40 years of age = 180 MHR

180 MHR x .60 = 108 180 MHR x .70 = 126

Target Heart Rate for Fat Burning is 108-126

For session with low intensity, long duration aerobic activity you want to stay in your THR Zone (60-70%) for exercise periods of 45 minutes to 1 hour. This gives you plenty of time to get into the Krebs Cycle. Remember, the Krebs Cycle is not at its maximum energy production until for a minimum of at least 16 – 20 minutes in any significant amount.) As a rough guide of intensity you should be able to carry on a light, clipped conversation during this activity.

The second type of aerobic activity is the higher intensity shorter duration variety. This type uses intervals, alternating between higher and lower intensities. Using the formula for Max HR already shown, your intention is to exercise at 90% of MHR for 1 – 2 minutes then back off and exercise at 50% of MHR for 1 – 2 minutes. This type of exercise burns more overall calories, and keeps your metabolism ramped up longer after the activity has ended. Eventually, you can alternate back and forth between intensities for 20 – 30 minutes.

As already noted, both types of aerobic intensities have their place in the fat burning regimen. Whereas, the lower intensity, longer duration session burns a greater % of fat calories, it is a larger % of an overall smaller number. Higher intensity, interval type training burns more carbohydrates because there are times of low or no oxygen, a greater number of calories are burned albeit a lower % of fat calories. I know that this is a little confusing so the chart below illustrates this point a little clearer.

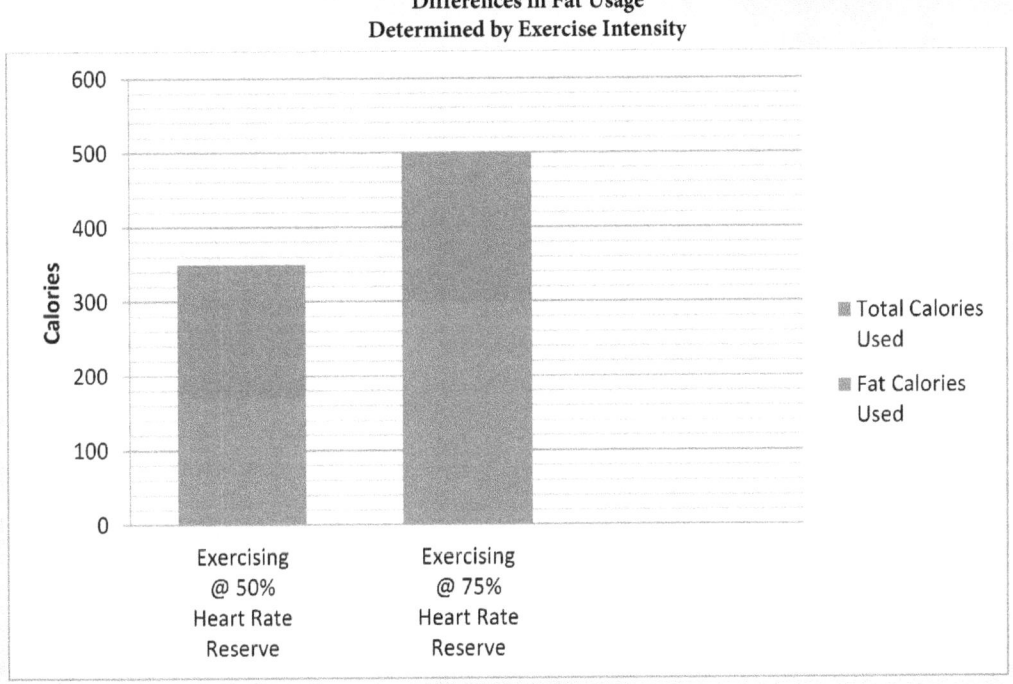

As you can determine from the chart, exercising at 50% of Heart Rate Reserve uses 50% fat calories for every calories used as energy, whereas, exercising at 75% of Heart Rate Reserve uses only 40% fat calories for every calorie used as energy. So even though the %'s are greater exercising at a lower intensity, performing the activity for approximately 30 minutes at each intensity, you will use more overall fat calories exercising at the higher intensity.

Goals	Straight Line % Max HR	Karvonen % HRR	Rate of Perceived Exertion	Adaptations
Trains the body to burn fat	60-70%	50-65%	3-4	Increase fat utilization, aerobic energy sources, pathways, capillaries, mitochondria and free fatty acid mobilization
Endurance Gains	70-75%	65-75%	4-6	Increase Aerobic Energy Sources and Pathways
Endurance / Strength Gains	75-80%	75-80%	6-7	Increase Aerobic Pathways, Increase Aerobic Glycolysis, Increase FOG fiber usage, oxygen transport system
Lactate Threshold	80-90%	80-90%	7-8	Increase lactate threshold, aerobic and anaerobic energy pathways, oxygen transport
Fast Peak	90-100%	90-100%	9-10	Increase anaerobic energy sources, fast twitch fiber recruitment

Adapted from Sleamaker R, 1989. Serious Training for Endurance Athletes. 2nd Edition Champaign, IL; Human Kinetics p.60

TIME

The duration of cardiovascular exercise is dependent on which type of exercise you perform and at what intensity you are performing them. In order to enter the Krebs cycle you need to be exercising 16 minutes or longer, however if you are exercising at a high enough intensity and using enough overall muscle, then you can use a shorter duration to perform the same amount of overall work.

TYPE / MODE

The answer to what type of cardio should be attempted is simple - What do you like to do, and what will you do consistently. Large muscles use more overall calories, so running or jogging would definitely be a good start. Bicycling is also good, but get outside and ride an outdoor bike in lieu of an exercise bike or recumbent bike at your gym. Remember, we want more overall muscles used. Swimming is not very effective at getting lean. Once you are lean, swimming definitely can help you remain muscle tone, but overall, you will not burn enough calories in the pool. People with more fat stores are more buoyant and give up less heat in the water - thus fewer calories are burned or given up as energy.

In addition to determining what mode of exercise you will consistently perform, you must also determine what type of Cardiovascular Program you will employ and how it matches up with your goals.

Types of Cardiovascular / Aerobic Programs

Type	Characteristics
Continuous Rhythmic	Steady State Aerobics normally performed for longer periods of time
Interval Training	Using Pre-Established Timed Intervals to perform work
Fartlek Training	Alternating Fast and Slow Intensity
Cross Training	Using sports or activities outside of major activity to accomplish cardiovascular fitness

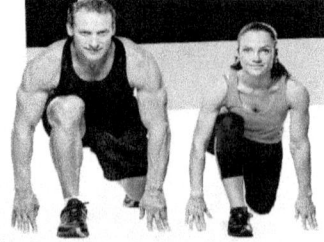

Specific Modes of Cardiovascular / Aerobic

Jogging

This is a very popular form of cardiovascular exercise with a quick learning curve. It is relatively inexpensive (the only thing needed is a decent pair of running shoes) and it can be done virtually anywhere. One potential drawback is the body seems to adapt very quickly to this mode of exercise. This means that if you are not continually changing the stimuli, speed, distance or route taken your body will plateau or become more efficient at performing the same amount of work. Not recommended for fat loss.

Stair Stepper

The stair stepper has declined in popularity from its heyday when it first made the fitness scene, but it offers a great workout when done correctly. However, the majority of people training on these machines uses a very small range of motion and drape themselves over the ma-chine making it a very ineffective fat burner. You tend to work your calves at very high intensity levels, but not much of anything else when using this machine. Again the short range of motion already noted is not recommended.

Rowing Machine

History repeats itself. This machine has gone through cycles of popularity. This machine offers a non - impact workout while using both the upper and lower body. When performed correctly and gives some resistance training properties for select muscle group in the upper body.

Treadmill

The treadmill is a fixture in any gym or training center. You will see plenty of people using these things; however you will see very little change in their physiques because they don't push themselves "hard enough". They barely plod along at a snail's pace. When used correctly, and at a high enough intensity (through adjusting the speed and in-cline), this machine can be very effective tool for the war on fat.

ABSESSION

Elliptical Machine

This is one of the "it" machines in health clubs across America. The elliptical machine combines upper and lower body movements. Part cross country skiing, part bicycle, the arms move in a linear motion, while the lower body moves in an ellipsis. An added benefit surfaces when the lower body can go in both directions (forward and back-ward). This machine offers a full body workout and enhanced caloric expenditure by using multiple "big muscle groups." One of the greatest benefits of the elliptical machine is its non-impact nature on the body a big benefit for people with bad knees, hips or ankles who would be greatly aggravated by running.

Bicycling (stationary)

These bikes come in various shapes and models. Recumbent, Upright, and the now "all the rage" Spinning Bikes are currently marketed out there for the cycling enthusiasts. This does use the muscles of the lower body; however it doesn't use those muscles to maximum capacity. Basically, it only uses the smaller muscles of the lower body to a very high degree of intensity. Overall, a good calorie burner, but I would opt for the outdoor model of bike because it calls into play more overall muscle groups due to the additional factor of maintaining one's balance.

Cross Country Ski Machine

This is probably one of the greatest aerobic / cardiovascular activities anyone could perform for fat loss. It uses virtually every muscle in the body, while offering no impact on the joints. While the machine takes some accustomization, the operation is not difficult to master. This machine mimics the outdoor activity very closely and offers an overall body workout while enjoying a significant caloric expenditure.

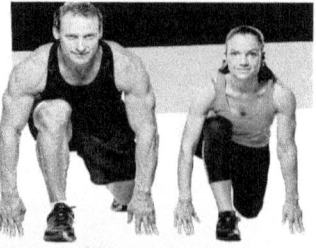

Step Mill / Stair Gauntlet

Picture a flight of stairs that goes on forever and you will have a rea-sonable image of this machine's operation. Adjustable speed makes it more challenging than just walking or running stairs, but just slightly. Once again, you are using fewer overall muscle at a very high inten-sity (re: lactic acid buildup) instead of using many muscles at a more moderate intensity (re: fat burner). Although, it does work the glutes and hamstrings well enough to be considered somewhat of a resis-tance exercise for the 2 bodyparts.

And there are many more …

Remember, the best form of cardiovascular / aerobic exercise is the one that you will perform consistently and routinely

If you notice all of these modes of exercise mentioned above have one thing in common, they all call big muscles into play. The more overall muscle is used the greater the amount of calories burned and the greater the amount of fat loss. **Remember one pound of fat is comprised of 3500 kcals.**

Kcals are what is most commonly referred to as calories. A calorie is a unit of measurement. It is the amount of energy it takes to increase the temperature of one liter of water one degree centigrade. More appropriately for our context, it is the amount of energy that is stored in food.

Once you start losing some of your spare tire or set of tires, and you experience a greater level of fitness, you will be ready to increase your intensity. It is not as easy as you think – you don't just crank up your percent of maximum heart rate to 95-100% that would be self – defeating. Rather, you will use what is called the Karvonen Formula and for that you will need to know your Resting Heart Rate (RHR).

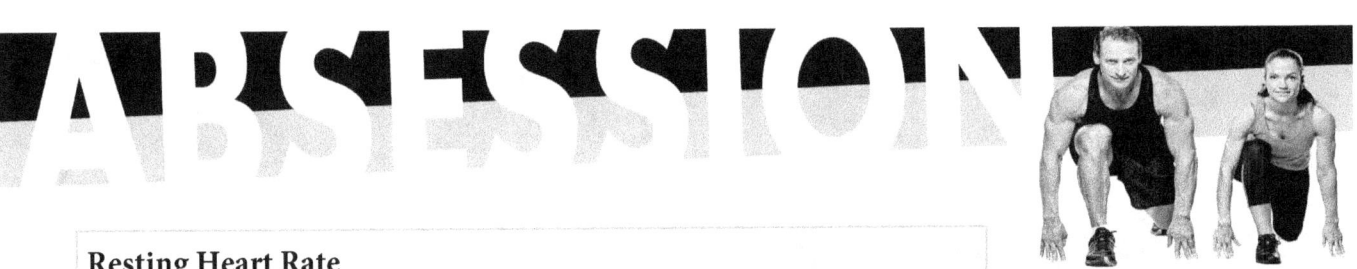

Resting Heart Rate

The clinical definition of resting heart rate (RHR) is the number of times your heart beats for one full minute, as soon as you open your eyes, before your feet hit the floor. As your level of fitness improves, your resting heart rate (RHR) will become lower, because your heart will become more efficient and won't have to perform as hard to conduct the same amount of work.

The Karvonen Formula takes into account your level of fitness, by using your RHR to calculate your target heart rate (THR). The formula is easy to use and it looks like this;

$$220 - Age = Max\ HR$$

$$Max\ HR - Resting\ Heart\ Rate = Heart\ Rate\ Reserve\ (HRR)$$

(Example; % for maximum fat utilization is 50-65% of HRR).

Once you determine your Maximum Heart Rate by subtracting your age from 220, then you want to subtract your Resting Heart Rate (RHR). This will give you what is called your Heart Rate Reserve (HRR). At this point you will take the % for intensity found on the preceding chart and multiply the % by the HRR. After multiplying you will add back in your RHR to determine your Target Heart Rate (THR). You will perform this for both the low end and the high end of the intensity levels for your desired bodily responses.

Although, the **Straight Line Method** works very well for beginners, the body is resilient enough to adapt very quickly to aerobic exercise. In order to continue achieving maximum gains, you must continually change the stimuli. One way to accomplish this is by accounting for your improved level of fitness via the **Karvonen Formula**.

Rate of Perceived Exertion (RPE) is a subjective, as opposed to objective way to monitor exercise intensity. You, the exerciser can assign an arbitrary number from 1-10 to subjectively rate your intensity. The parameters are graded from 1 to 10. The number one represents you at home sitting down watching television and ten represents you running for your life. The approximate level we are targeting in order to maintain optimum fat burning is 3-4.

Let me mention here that there are some inherent problems with RPE:

1) Again, it is subjective- if you are being a wuss, then it won't really work.

2) The 1-10 levels refer to your breathing and not any other maladies, injuries, aches or pains you may have. I personally don't care for this measuring parameter, although it has become increasingly popular among group fitness classes.

Another way to monitor intensity that mainly focuses on whether or not you are in a fat burning mode is the talk test. Remember back in Chapter One – Energy Systems? You need oxygen and water to break apart Triglycerides and oxygen means aerobics, or better put air.

The talk test states that you should be able to carry on a conversation in clipped sentences. If you labor so much you can't talk, you are exercising too hard. Conversely, if you can drone on and on without missing a beat or taking a breath, you are not exercising hard enough. At that point you need to pick up the pace a little bit!

Now that you know about the chemistry, intensity and the modes, it is appropriate to discuss the when. Just *when* do you perform your Aerobic / Cardiovascular Exercise to **<u>Maximize Fat Loss?</u>**

There are two schools of thought. The first concept states that a calorie is a calorie and 3500 **kcal = 1** pound of fat. Eliminate 3500 kcal a week through a sensible diet with exercise and no doubt you will lose weight. *Notice I said weight, not fat!* The second school of thought relies on the concept that the composition of the calories and the timing of the calories determine whether weight is lost or fat is lost. Since the layer or layers of flab are between you and your six pack, let's adopt this second school of thought and concern ourselves with losing fat as opposed to just losing weight. I know this sounds very obvious. However, weight loss could be attributed to other things than fat loss. Lean muscle tissue, muscle glycogen and even organ tissue could all contribute to overall weight loss. Our goal is to lose the flab and maintain any lean body tissue and this program will accomplish just that.

To achieve optimum fat loss, the most effective time to do your cardio is first thing early in the morning in a fasted state on an empty stomach. Here's why; during the course of the night, the body needs glucose to fuel the brain, heart and other vital organ functions. Once it depletes the glucose running through your blood the body will eventually taps into stored carbohydrates found in the liver. If you do aerobic exercise in a carb depleted state, with no blood glucose, in order to produce ATP, your body must seek out fat stores for energy provided the intensity is within the suggested %'s of Max HR.

I believe this is the most optimum and effective time to exercise and I make that suggestion to all of my clients. I strongly recommend they drink a cup of black coffee upon awakening then within the hour, hit their aerobic activity. After concluding their exercise they can refuel with a good breakfast.

Another advantageous opportunity to perform cardiovascular aerobic activity is "after" your resistance training session. Resistance training is anaerobic in nature. The major fuel source for anaerobic activities and resistance training in particular are carbohydrates, and more specifi-cally glucose and glycogen stored in muscle and liver. You are not going to burn much fat lifting weights. There is just too much stop and go activity. That is why you allow your nutrition and your cardiovascular / aerobic exercise to handle your fat stores. However, there is a benefit to combining your training sessions. If you perform your aerobic exercise **immediately after** you perform your resistance training, you will be in a carb depleted state. Remember, resistance training uses carbohydrates (glucose and glycogen) as an energy source, so that energy system will be lessened to a greater degree, allowing you to tap into fat stores more quickly.

Both ways of cardiovascular / aerobic exercise have their advantages and disadvantages, but they both do one thing--- they both help you incinerate **your body's fat stores!**

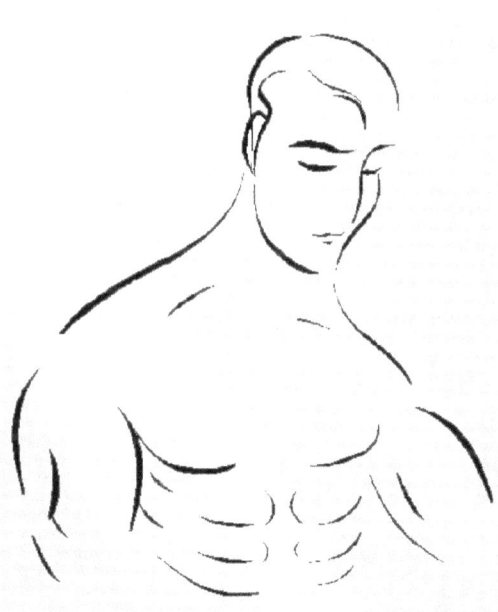

"If a man is weak of heart nothing else really matters…."

Unknown

ABSESSION

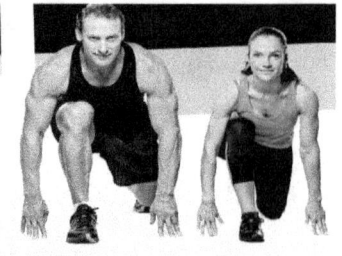

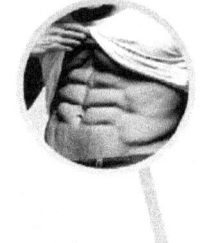

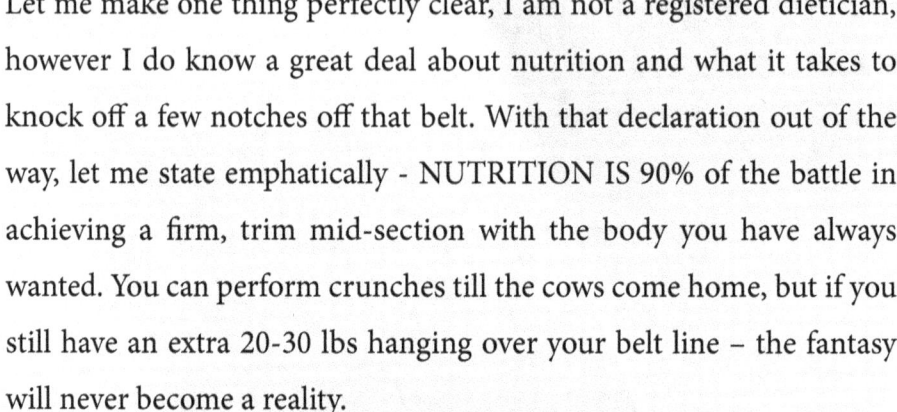

Let me make one thing perfectly clear, I am not a registered dietician, however I do know a great deal about nutrition and what it takes to knock off a few notches off that belt. With that declaration out of the way, let me state emphatically - NUTRITION IS 90% of the battle in achieving a firm, trim mid-section with the body you have always wanted. You can perform crunches till the cows come home, but if you still have an extra 20-30 lbs hanging over your belt line – the fantasy will never become a reality.

Total number of calories consumed vs. total number of calories exhausted determines whether you gain weight, lose weight or maintain your weight. The bigger piece of the puzzle lies in the composition of the calories consumed and the times at which you consume them, whether you lose fat or weight. This leads us naturally and logically into the discussion of diet!

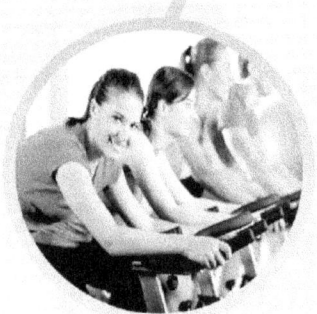

The word diet has a very negative connotation attached to it. Thoughts of self deprivation, starving oneself and having low energy and hunger pangs pervade our minds. In reality, the word DIET comes to us from the Greek and means **"Way of Life"**. I feel if we moved back to this original meaning of "Way of Life" and the accompanying philosophy of moderation in everything, we would not have the obesity epidemic that is plaguing America. Current statistics state that over 70% of adults and over 50% of children will be clinically obese by the year 2012.

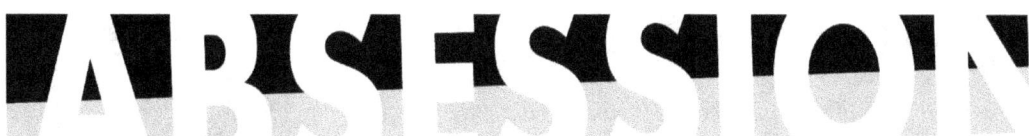
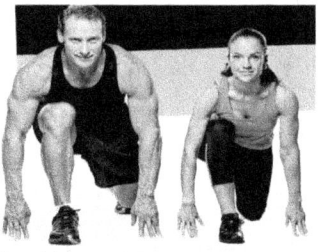

Furthermore, experts have predicted that obesity will soon be the number one preventable reason for death, surpassing smoking.

> **"Remember We Eat to Live, We Don't Live to Eat"**

Just as crude oil is refined to produce gasoline for our vehicles, the food we eat is refined to produce energy for our bodies. Just as your car won't go very far on an empty tank, your body needs fuel to live life, albeit not too much at any one time.

The food we eat is comprised of Macronutrients and Micronutrients. Just as their names imply; **Macronutrients** are the nutrients we need in large quantities and Micronutrients are the nutrients we need in small quantities. Macronutrients include: Carbohydrates, Protein, and Fats. The Micronutrients are comprised of Minerals and Vitamins. The forgotten nutrient (as I call it) is water. The body needs water in large quantities. It is the medium by which all life sustaining metabolic functions take place within the body (more on this later).

The first macronutrient and the most maligned is the Carbohydrate. Carbohydrates have been blamed for everything from obesity to Type II Diabetes. However, Carbohydrates are the preferred source of energy pressuring the body to do whatever it can to make sure it has adequate glucose and glycogen stores. It will even tap into a protein source to fuel the body. This less than advantageous redirection process is called Gluconeogenesis, but more on this later. When you are resistance training, the consumption of an adequate amount of Carbs is imperative to your success.

Once carbohydrates are ingested, they move from the stomach into the small intestines to be broken down into simple sugars by amylase an enzyme that specifically targets carbs. Those simple sugars are then transported from the intestines into the blood as glucose. If you recall I said that carbohydrates come in two styles; Simple and Complex. Simple Carbs are broken down into glucose more preferentially over complex carbohydrates.

Simple Carbohydrates come in 2 forms; Monosaccharide and Disaccharides. Monosaccharides contain one sugar bond linking glucose and fructose, while disaccharides contain two sugar bonds linking fructose, dextrose and sucrose.

Complex Carbohydrates come in Polysaccharides and Fibers which are both soluble and insoluble. Fiber, particularly insoluble fiber is **not** digestible. Insoluble fiber absorbs water from the small intestines then uses this hydration process to easily excrete waste. An inadequate intake of insoluble fiber inhibits the body's ability to discard waste products.

A more effective way to manage your carbohydrates and ultimately your insulin levels is to monitor the glycemic index of the foods you eat. The glycemic index (GI) was originally a rating system devised for diabetics to monitor blood glucose levels. The GI assigns a value to foods strictly based on how quickly 100 grams of Carbs make your blood glucose level raise. Food with a higher assigned GI value will consistently cause a more rapid spike in insulin. This spiking effect is not advisable and can be avoided by combining macronutrients, high GI foods with lower GI foods.

Foods with a glycemic index (GI) of less than 55 are considered low glycemic indexed foods. Some examples of low glycemic foods include; Oatmeal, Brown Rice, Legumes and Apples. These foods are digested more slowly and cause a gradual increase in blood glucose levels.

ABSESSION

The polar opposite of low glycemic foods are high glycemic foods. High glycemic foods have a glycemic index of 70 or higher and are digested very quickly causing a spike in blood glucose levels. Some examples of high glycemic indexed foods are: white bread, table sugar, pre sweetened breakfast cereals and some pasta. The chart below further illustrates the glycemic index of some commonly eaten foods.

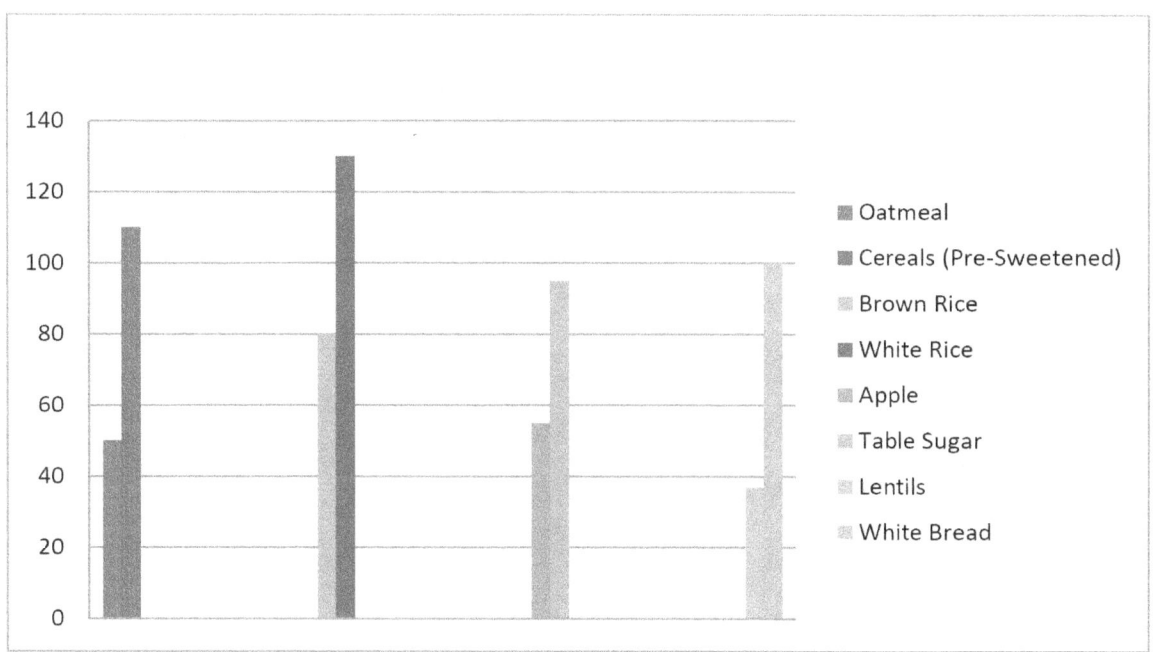

I want to stress that the glycemic index of a food is basically determined by how quickly blood sugar rises after consumption. The question is; what determines how fast a food affects a spike in blood sugar levels? There are several factors that determine a food's GI:

- Amount of processing the food has undergone
- Type of carbohydrate (s) the food contains
- Any additional macronutrients that comprise the food
- Amount of fiber in the food
- Type of grain(s) that reside in the food

Low glycemic foods are more natural foods; they contain complex Carbs, normally have more fiber, contain additional macronutrients other than Carbs and come from less refined grains.

You can obtain a complete food list with their corresponding GI values at Mendosa.com.

High glycemic foods are not always villainous. The sole time the consumption of higher glyce-mic foods can be advantageous is immediately after resistance training. The coupling of a complete protein and a high glycemic carbohydrate will enable you to take advantage of a natural insulin spike enabling you to start the repair process.

High glycemic foods are not always villainous. The sole time the consumption of higher glyce-mic foods can be advantageous is immediately after resistance training. The coupling of a complete protein and a high glycemic carbohydrate will enable you to take advantage of a natural insulin spike enabling you to start the repair process.

Insulin is a hormone that is secreted by the pancreas in order to remove and store unsafe amounts of glucose from the blood stream. Here is an example, after consuming a heavy carbohydrate meal, the body breaks down the food into glucose. Blood sugar levels are measured in deciliters per millimeter of blood. Normal glucose ranges are 80-100 deciliters per milliliter. When your glucose levels rise above this level it is referred to as hyperglycemic. The body constantly fights for a point of leveling or homeostasis (evenness) and will release the hormone insulin to remove the glucose from the blood. Glucose will then be stored in one of three places; 1) Liver, 2) Muscle or 3) FAT!! Both the liver and the muscle are relatively resistant to absorbing the glucose quickly, but the body's FAT stores are more than willing and able to hoard this quick moving glucose. However, there a critical moment when you can take advantage of the body's naturally occurring insulin that is immediately after resistance training.

Let me explain. After resistance training, your muscle cell receptor sites are active. In order to start the repair process, you need to supply carbohydrates with protein which has been broken down into its building blocks of amino acids. A spike in insulin, caused by the consumption of higher glycemic carbohydrates will remove the glucose from the blood and along with it the amino acids. Assuming you have worked out hard enough, the muscle cell receptor sites are now engorged and depleted of muscle glycogen and insulin will drive the glucose and the amino acids back into the muscle initiating the repair process. This would be the only time

I would advise eating higher glycemic carbohydrates to reduce body fat. Most other times, a lower glycemic carbohydrate will do nicely.

According to experts, controlling blood sugar levels and insulin levels is vital for basic health reasons not just fat loss. Heart disease, colon and other certain types of cancers, Alzheimer's disease and Type II Diabetes, are life threatening ailments partly controlled by a proper diet.

As a general rule, here are some sound strategies to use hormonal insulin in your own,

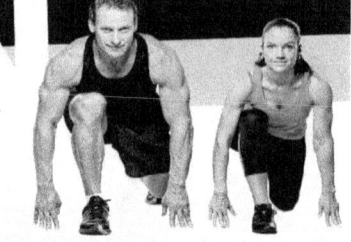

ABSESSION

Regulating Insulin Levels to Maximize Fat Loss

1. Eat Carbs over 5-6 Meals, Not all in one sitting.

2. Eat Plenty of Soluble Fiber.

3. Vegetables, Vegetables, Vegetables.

4. Consume Protein with each meal.

5. Consume Omega 3 Fatty Acids.

6. Say no to Saturated Fats, they desensitize muscle fibers to insulin.

7. Consume the majority of Carbs at Breakfast, Pre-Post Workout.

8. Limit Simple Carbs to Post Workout.

Protein is probably the most misunderstood macronutrient. Protein is vital and structurally important in the repair of muscle tissue, skin, hair, nails etc. However, the current belief seems to be, "the more the better." Eating obscene amounts of protein does not produce increased muscle mass, resistance training does! Protein, like other food group will eventually come to a fork in the road to be burned in a biological system or stored in one as fat. As already mentioned, if you ingest too few carbohydrates protein will be converted to glucose via a process called Gluconeogenesis.

Once protein is ingested it makes its way to the small intestine. It is here that the enzyme pepsin breaks down the protein into its smaller amino acids building blocks.

Your body requires twenty amino acids for normal, healthy functioning derived from the breakdown of its parent protein source. Whereas, carbohydrates come in simple and complex forms, protein comes in two varieties, a complete form containing all twenty amino acids and an incomplete form containing some amino acids. Your body can and does make some amino acids but not all. These are referred to as non-essential, because they do not require an external source. But many can only be extracted from the food you eat. They are referred to as essential amino acids. In order for protein to effectively repair muscle tissue, all of the twenty camion acids must be present.

3 Amino Acids make up approximately 60% of all muscle tissue. So, for those concerned about adding lean muscle mass and ridding yourself of that mid-section flab the 3 most important amino acids that can help are the branched chain amino acids; valine, leucine and isoleucine.

Amino Acids are used not only to build and repair protein based muscle tissue, they also regenerate new skin cells, assists in the synthesization of hormones and enzymes, and synthesizes hair and nail proteins.

The following are some important points to remember about protein as it relates to training:

- Resistance and Cardiovascular Training Programs do increase the body's protein demand.

- Active people should consume 1.4 to 2.0 gram of protein per kilogram of body-weight per day.

- When protein is part of a balanced diet there has been no direct correlation between increased protein consumption and impaired kidney function.

- Consumption of protein before and after training increases the rate of muscle recovery and moves the body's biochemistry out of a state of catabolism into an anabolic state.

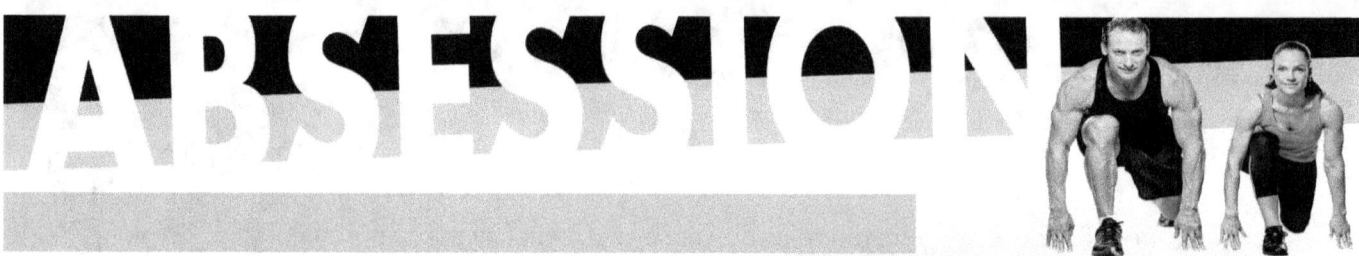

When dietary fats are ingested, they move from the stomach to the small intestine where they are broken down into free fatty acids (FFA's) by the enzyme lipase. Fat is carried throughout the body in the blood by the emulsifier bile. Dietary fat is divided into 3 classifications: Saturated, Monounsaturated and Polyunsaturated.

Saturated fats are easy to spot; they are hard at room temperature and chemically raise serum cholesterol. They are definitely not healthy for you. Monounsaturated fats are liquid at room temperature, have no effect on serum cholesterol levels. Polyunsaturated fatty acids are liquid at room temperature and come in omega 6 varieties, predominantly found in plants and Omega 3 varieties, present mostly in fish. The polyunsaturated have a varying effect on cholesterol and triglyceride levels.

Fat serves several purposes in the body:

- Dietary fat allows "fat soluble" vitamins A,D,E,K to be absorbed in the body.

- Dietary fat is a precursor to prostaglandins.

- Fats are necessary for healthy skin.

- Monounsaturated fats may improve serum cholesterol levels.

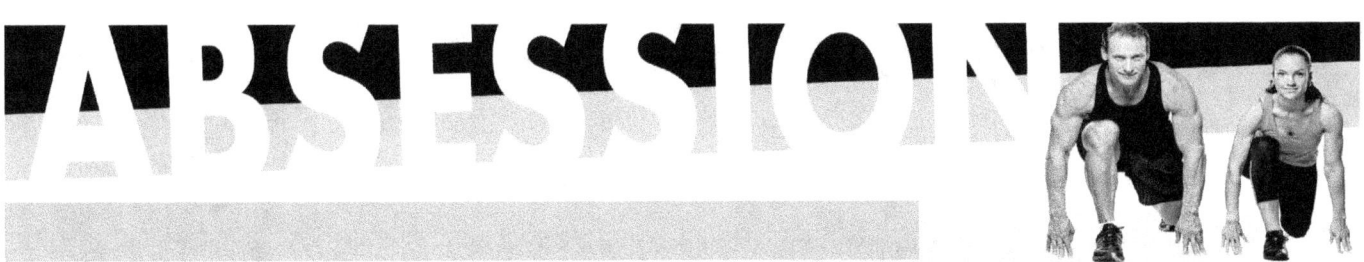

Since we are talking about fats, we should naturally talk about cholesterol. Cholesterol is basically the fat in your blood, and body cells. You know what happens when you put fat in water-in floats. So in order for cholesterol to be transported in the water based blood serum it needs a transporter. That transporter is called a lipoprotein.

A lipoprotein wraps itself around cholesterol so it can be transported in the aqueous blood. Lipoproteins come in basically two types: Low density lipoprotein (LDL) and High density lipoprotein (HDL).

Low Density Lipoproteins (LDL's) are considered bad cholesterol transporters. Because they do such a poor transport job, too high a level of LDL's can lead to coronary disease. High Density Lipoproteins (HDL's) are considered good cholesterol transporters. HDL's carry cholesterol away from vital organs and escort it to the liver for excretion. Regular cardiovascular exercise increases HDL's and reduce the likelihood of coronary heart disease.

Trans-fatty acids are the "new kid on the block" when it comes to dietary fat. Trans fatty acids are man-made and are very prevalent in most food not located on the outer rim of the supermarket. Next time you visit a supermarket eye the outer rim of the market; Vegetables, Dairy, Meats, Whole Grains. Food manufacturers fill their products snack, fast food, and convenience food items with trans fatty acids to extend shelf life. These Tran fatty acids are the "by products" of the process called hydrogenation.

Hydrogenation was discovered and judiciously brought to us chiefly by the fast-food industry. They realized that by hydrogenation, cooking grease could be stretched and develop "more mileage" (more batches of french fries) for every vat of grease.

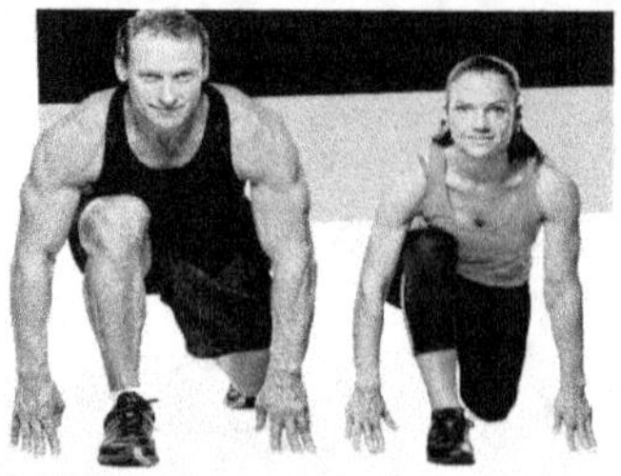

Studies have shown that the ingestion of trans fatty acids lead to abdominal obesity, high blood pressure, increased risk of Type II Diabetes, increased risk of stroke, hyperlipidemia and a host of other health maladies.

Foods that Contain Healthy Fats

- Almonds
- Tuna
- Salmon
- Mackerel
- Olive Oil
- Walnuts
- Cashews
- Peanuts
- Eggs

Food that Contain Unhealthy Fats

- Fried Foods
- Butter
- Coconut Oil
- Red Meats that aren't lean

Water is the medium for just about every biochemical and cellular reaction taking place in your body. It assists in the transportation of glucose in the blood, eliminates waste products, helps cool the body and here's a big one, it comprises 70% of muscle. Dehydration can impair all of these processes and many others. Severe dehydration can lead to serious health complication and in the worst case scenario, even death.

While training, you should drink water before, during and after activity. Do not allow thirst to determine when you consume water. By the time you reach that limit of thirst, you are already too low. The best indicator of hydration levels is reflected in the color and frequency of your urine. Normal frequency with clear color suggests a normal water balance. If your urine is dark and below a reasonable volume, you are probably below normal water balance levels.

The usual recommendation for water ingestion is a minimum of 8 – 8 oz. glasses of water everyday. On hot or active days or exercising, this is probably not enough. For exercisers, and those looking to reduce body fat, I would suggest taking 2/3 of your body weight in ounces of water per day. Below is a formula to determine your daily water recommendations.

Body Weight _____ pounds x .66 = _____ ounces of water per day

Micronutrients are those nutrients required only in small or trace amounts. Vitamins and Minerals fall into this category.

Vitamins and Minerals **DO NOT PROVIDE ENERGY!!!!** There are no calories in a vitamin or a mineral. However, vitamins and minerals are important because they are co-factors that regulate biochemical and cellular reactions in the body. They work in conjunction with enzymes to effect biochemical reactions in the body, changing one molecule into another or joining molecules together. Vitamins and Minerals do not increase performance; however a deficiency can lead to a decline in performance and health.

In a perfect world, that is when dependably eating a well balanced diet - you would normally ingest sufficient amounts of vitamins and minerals. Recommendations currently hold that a multi-vitamin would be enough to supplement any deficiencies in your diet.

A free is an unstable molecule. This instability is caused by the lack of an electron in its chemical structure. The free radical will then "borrow" or better put "steal" an electron from a stable molecule, creating a "new free radical". This domino effect occurs over and over again, until the free radical either combines with a single electron molecule or the process is brought to a screeching halt by an anti-oxidant. The problem with free radicals is they are very dangerous and very destructive. They attack protein, carbohydrates, lipids and have even been known to attack DNA and RNA strands. They specifically target and attack unsaturated lipids located on the cell membranes.

The good news is that anti oxidants neutralize free radicals. This is done by changing the free radicals into a less ominous form – hydrogen peroxide. Anti oxidants prevent oxidative damage to the body's cells. Some of this oxidative damage does occur as a result of resistance training. This damage, if left unchecked can lead to a host of health problems. These maladies include; cancers, heart disease, diabetes, cataracts and even autoimmune diseases. Anti-oxidants found in multi vitamins are also important because they control the actions of free radicals that lead to oxidation that are produced by exercise. Free radicals have been accused of speeding up the aging process, but in reality they slow down the normal biochemical reactions in the body that are constructive in nature.

The great news is it is easy to find "whole foods" that contain the anti oxidants needed to protect free radicals. Some great sources are;

The following are some basic nutritional recommendations: This breakdown scheme represents a ratio profile of the total amount of calories you consume each day. You may need to adjust this balance to meet your own individual dietary needs and goals (Refer to Figure 3.2).

- 60% Carbohydrates - Current research suggests that no more than 10% may be in the form of simple sugars. People training should target 6-10 grams per kilogram of bodyweight.

- 25% Protein - This percentage should be evaluated in relationship to ingesting 1.4 – 1.8 grams / kg bodyweight per day and adjusted accordingly.

- 15% Fats – With no more than 5% should be in the form of saturated fat.

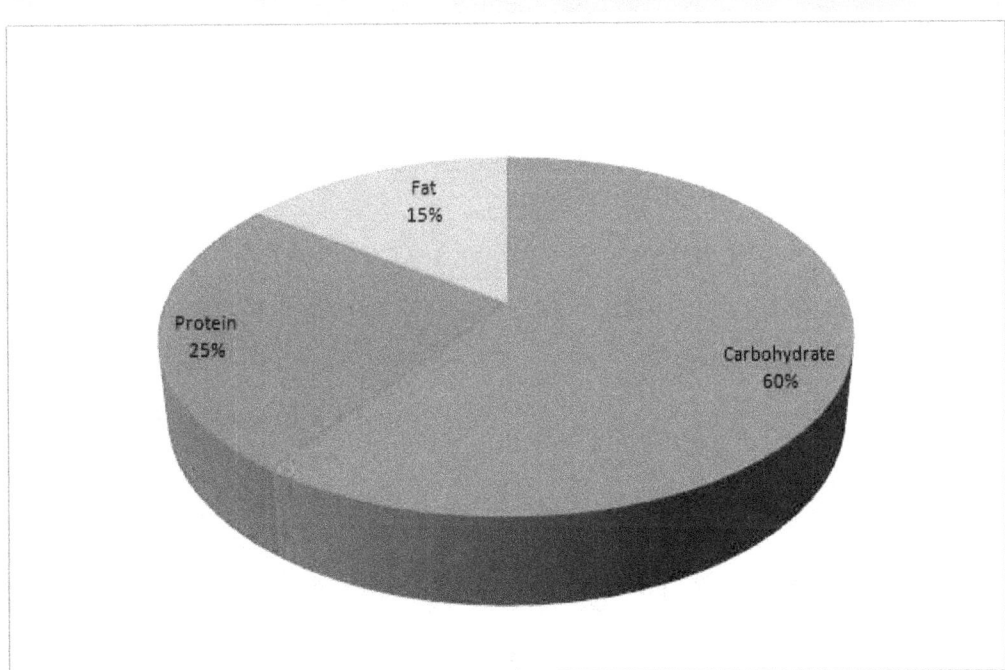

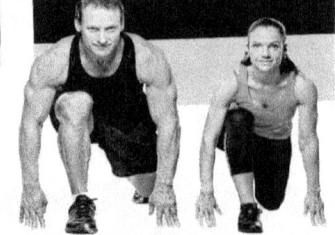

Recommendations for Fat Loss

1. Eat More Often

   5-6 meals a day will keep insulin levels in check while supplying amino acids to your muscles, thus keeping you in an anabolic and not catabolic state.

2. Minimize Simple or Refined Carbohydrates

   Post workout meals should be the only time simple carbs are consumed, thus taking advantage of the body's natural production of insulin to drive nutrients back into muscle cells.

3. Load the front end of your meals

   Breakfast and lunch must be your largest meals. Your body naturally starts to "slow down" as evening approaches, as day turns to night calories have a greater opportunity to be stored as body fat due to your reduction in activity.

4. Minimize Saturated and Hydrogenated Fats

   Studies have shown that both of these types of fats lead to a greater risk of coronary disease and should be consumed sparingly.

5. Do not skip Breakfast

   Breakfast is exactly what is says; "Breaking the fast from the previous night". Your body uses up glucose and glycogen stores during the night for vital body functions, skipping breakfast can lead to a state of hypoglycemia.

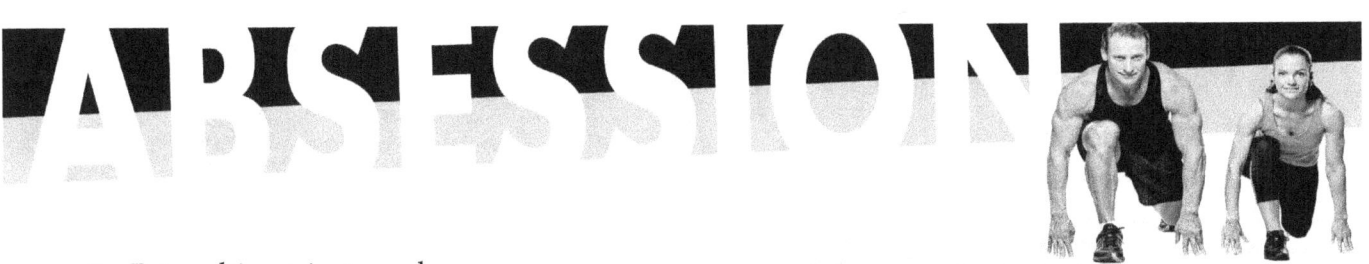

6. Eat multi nutrient meals

Your plate should resemble a peace symbol. A protein source, a starch source and a vegetable source. Remember "Man does not live by protein alone".

7. Eat Fiber

Most fiber has what is termed a net effect. Which means it takes more energy (calories) to metabolize, than it possesses in calories.

8. On a satiety scale of 1 to 10, eat only to a level of a 7.

Your body has to catch up with your mind. If you eat only to a 7 on the "fullness" scale, you will be satisfied instead of being stuffed.

9. Eat slower

Eating too quickly will actually cause you to eat more because you will continue to eat until your body catches up with your head.

10. Choose low glycemic foods over high glycemic foods

Remember low glycemic foods cause a gradual raise in blood glucose levels, leading to less of those calories being shuttled into fat stores.

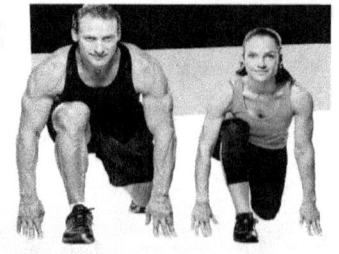

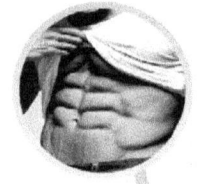

Before we can start putting together our resistance training portion of this program we must get acquainted with the muscles of the body and how they work. There are over 600 muscles in the human body and many are vital to achieve success in your training program. Yes, by the title of this chapter, you've got it – Anatomy and Physiology of muscles. We are going to examine muscle structure then review the major muscles of the body, their functions and their location. Let's take a look at just how muscles contract, how they move against a resistance.

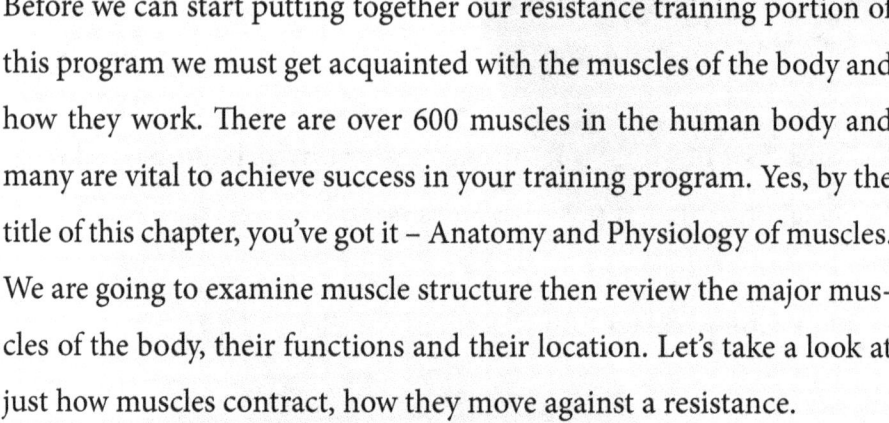

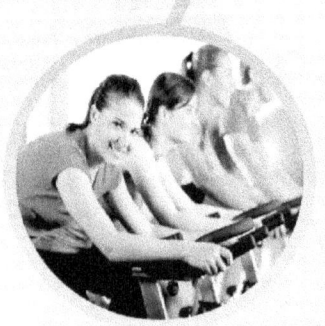

Muscles come in 3 distinct types; Smooth, Cardiac and Skeletal. Smooth muscle, also known as visceral muscle, is the muscle that lines the internal walls of vital organs. Cardiac muscle is the muscle that comprises the heart. Skeletal muscle, the most commonly thought of is the muscle that is attached to bones by tendons and when voluntarily contracted causes movement by pulling against bones. Muscles have two points at which they are attached to bone. One end, more stationary and usually closer to the mid-line of the body is called the origin. The opposite end of the muscle that is at the end where more movement occurs is called the insertion. Muscles work by pulling against bones, the muscle is a pulley of sorts, the bone a level working concurrently to produce movement.

All skeletal muscle is composed of small protein - like fibers. Of three generally accepted kinds, all 3 types of fibers exist in all skeletal muscle in varying ratios, determined largely by genetics and are marginally affected by the type of training one does.

The 3 muscle fibers types that comprise skeletal muscle are Type I known as Slow Twitch fibers or Red Fibers, Type II B, known as Fast Twitch or White Fibers, and Type IIA, known as Fast Oxidative Glycolytic Fibers or otherwise known as F.O.G. Fibers. These fibers have different properties and are stimulated in different ways requiring different stimuli to experience hypertrophy or more simply put, muscle growth due to contraction.

The smallest part of the muscle fiber is called the myofibril. Skeletal muscle is comprised of contractile proteins: Actin, Myosin, Troponin, and Tropomyosin. These contractile proteins grow larger through resistance training and subsequently continue to grow via rest and proper nutrition following resistance training.

The myofibril contains the contractile proteins that comprise skeletal muscle. The more myofibrilla a person has the greater his or her strength.

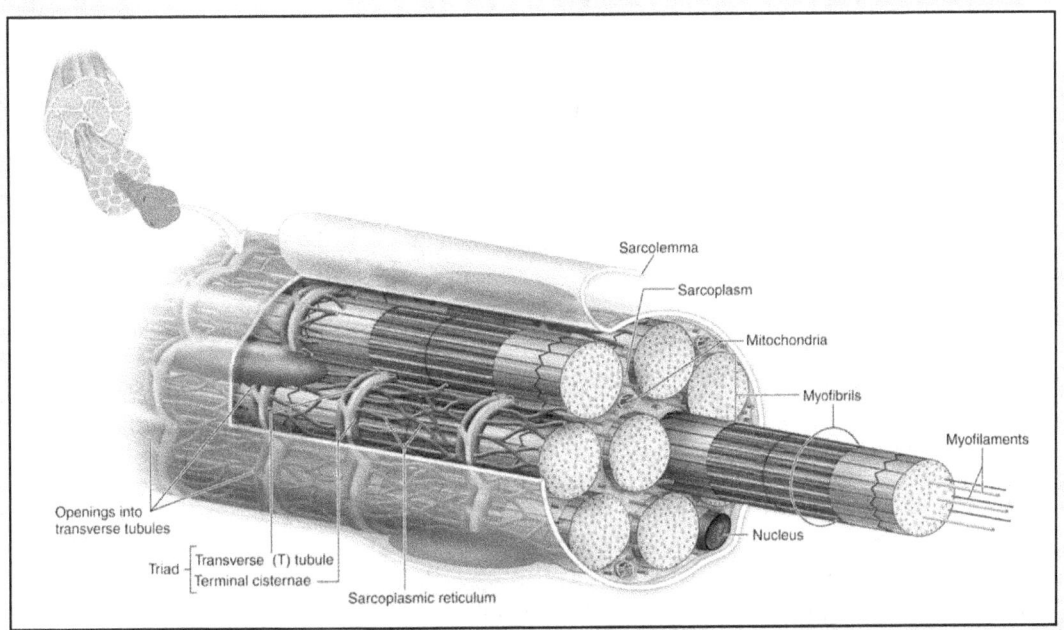

If you were to take a section of muscle (also known as a muscle biopsy) and examine it closely under a microscope, it would reveal the components that comprise skeletal muscle. Skeletal muscle is comprised primarily of water and contractile proteins. An easy way to illustrate the anatomical structure of muscle is to envision a coaxial cable that you may have hooked up to your television. If you were to cut through the coaxial cable you would see many smaller wires grouped together within the larger cable. This same set-up holds true for skeletal muscle. Muscle fibers are grouped together into a fasciculus by a covering known as an epimysium. A grouping of fasciculi is held together by the perimysium and smaller still the group of myofi-brils are held together by the endomysium. See Figure 5.1.

Through Gradual Progressive Resistance Training, the cross section of the contractile proteins will grow larger in size. This is called muscle hypertrophy. Muscle hypertrophy accounts for the majority of muscle size increase. Hyperplasia or the splitting of one fiber into 2 or more fibers is a theory that accounts for less than 10% of gains in musculature. Figure 4.2 summarizes muscle types and characteristics.

TYPE IIB WHITE	TYPE IIA (F.O.G.) PINK	TYPE I RED
FAST TWITCH	MEDIUM	SLOW TWITCH
GREAT ABILITY FOR GROWTH	MODERATE GROWTH	LIMITED ABILITY FOR GROWTH
LITTLE ENDURANCE	MODERATE ENDURANCE	GREAT ENDURANCE
GREAT POWER	MODERATE POWER	LIMITED POWER
GREAT CONTRACTION SPEED	MODERATE SPEED	LIMITED CONTRACTION SPEED
HIGH INTENSITY	MODERATE INTENSITY	LOW INTENSITY
THICK IN SIZE	MODERATE IN SIZE	THIN IN SIZE
ENERGY SYSTEM MAINLY ATP/CP SYSTEM	ENERGY SYSTEM ANAEROBIC GLYCOLYS	ENERGY SYSTEM BETA OXI-DATION
RESISTANCE TRAINING STIMULI 4-6 /8 REPS *	RESISTANCE TRAINING STIMULI 8-12 REPS *	RESISTANCE TRAINING STIMULI 12-15 AND UP REPS *

The ratio of fiber types that you possess significantly contribute to the kind of body type you possess. Your somatotype (a fancy way of saying body type) is one of three major classifications, ectomorph, mesomorph and endomorph. Most individuals are a combination of two out of the three somatotypes.

The ectomorph is the natural skinny and lean individual. The ectomorph has trouble putting on weight at all – whether it is fat or muscle. Ectomorphs have a very fast and or high metabolism. Narrow shoulders and narrow waists make up this person's physique.

The other end of the somatotype spectrum is the endomorph. Endomorphs are the naturally chubby person. They carry a great deal of body fat and they can add weight easily - both muscle and fat. Endomorphs have wide set hips, narrow shoulders, have a naturally slow metabolism and are shaped more like a pear.

The mesomorph is the body type everybody desires; yet few have. Wide shoulder and thin waists are the calling cards of this body type. Mesomorphs gain muscle easily and tend to carry very low levels of body fat.

The idea of someone fitting neatly into one of these somatotypes is rare. Normally, you find that people usually carry traits of two somatotypes. You will find Endo-Meso, or Meso-Ecto, but you will not find the two extreme combinations – Ecto-Endo. When determining your somato- type, think back to your body type when you were 18-20 years of age, before poor nutritional choices and a sedentary lifestyle derailed you. Unless you were naturally a skinny kid, a fat kid or a naturally buffed and muscular kid, you are probably a combination of 2 body types.

Here is a list of muscle groups and the function that are present in everyone regardless of somatotype...

Muscle Group	Muscles that Comprise Group	Action / Function
Chest	Pectoralis Major & Pectoralis Minor	Extension of arm, Horizontal Flexion, Adduction, and Internal Rotation of the humerus bone
Back	Trapezius I Trapezius II Trapezius III Latissimus Dorsi Rhomboids Erector Spinae	Elevate/Upwardly Rotate Scapula Retracts Scapula Depresses Scapula Extends, Adducts Arm Retracts Scapula, Elevates Shoulder Extends Spine, Rotates Trunk
Shoulders	Deltoid Anterior Deltoid Poster Deltoid Medial	Abducts Arm Extension of Shoulder Adducts Arm
Abdominals	Rectus Abdominis	Flexes Trunk & lower back stabilization
Biceps	Briceps Brachii Brachialis Brachioradialis	Flexes & Supinates Forearm Flexes Forearm
Triceps	Triceps Brachii	Extends Forearm
Quadriceps Group	Vastus Medialis Vastus Intermedius Vastus Lateralis Rectus Femoris	Extends Leg Flexes Hip & Extends Leg
Hamstrings	Bicep Femoris Semiteninosus Semimembranosus	Extends Hip & Flexes Leg
Calf	Gastrocnemius Soleus	Plantar flexes foot

The muscle contraction process begins with a nerve impulse traveling from the brain to the nerve involved. A motor nerve and all of the muscle fibers that it innervates is referred to as a motor unit. During muscle activation calcium is released from the sarcoplasmic reticulum and in particular the T Tubules. Next the calcium bonds with the contractile protein Troponin, pulls Tropomyosin out from between the Actin and Myosin contractile myofilamints. Once the Tropomyosin is removed, the myosin filament (the thicker filament) crosses over and makes contact with the Actin filament (the thinner filament). This is known as cross bridging. From there the swiveling heads located on the myosin are cocked and pivot causing the Actin filament to slide across the myosin. This is referred to as the **sliding filament theory.**

This process happens hundreds and thousands of times across the entire muscle fiber. As this happens the fibers contract and shorten (Picture a row of dominos knocked from both ends in towards the middle). This is known as **fiber bundling.**

This above listed process happens again and again, over and over during each repetition of a set. Some of the physiologic adaptations to resistance training can be found on the following chart.

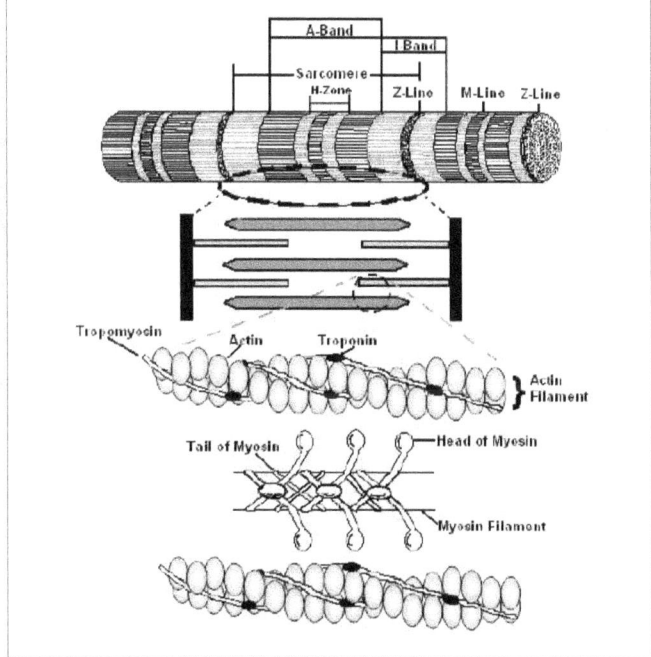

Your body responds and adapts to exercise in very specific ways, constantly searching for a point of homeostasis (which means "stability or balance"), so it responds to any training stimuli to avoid an unstable state. Some of the specific adaptations your body goes through exercising are found on the following chart.

Health Benefits / Postulated Health Benefits from Exercise

Rising Effects	Lowering Effects
Improves Blood Pressure Control	Lowers mortality rates for all ages
Increases High Density Lipoproteins	Decreases risk of cardiovascular disease
Improves Glucose tolerance	Decrease serum triglycerides
Improves overall health	Reduces insulin needs
Enhances feeling of well being	Decreases Risk of colon cancer
Enhances work, recreation performance	Lowers risk of Type II Diabetes
	Reduces resting systolic and diastolic blood-pressure
	Reduces Body Fat distribution
	Minimizes risk and effects of osteoporosis
	Relieves symptoms of depression, anxiety and -improves mood

* Adapted from the 1996 Surgeon General's Report

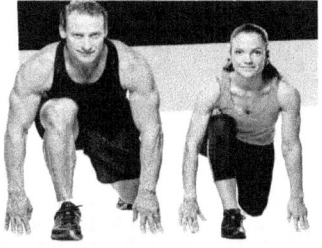

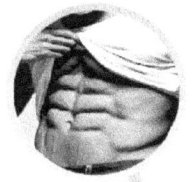

Resistance training is defined as activity that requires the body to move its levers against a resistance. Resistance Training can involve moving anything that offers resistance; no matter how that form of resistance comes. Machines, Free Weights, Jugs of Water, Even an immovable object. Performing resistance training is important in shedding body fat and uncovering your long awaited abdominal muscles. Gradual Progressive Overloading of the skeletal muscle causes adaptation. The body responds by making the skeletal muscle bigger and stronger.

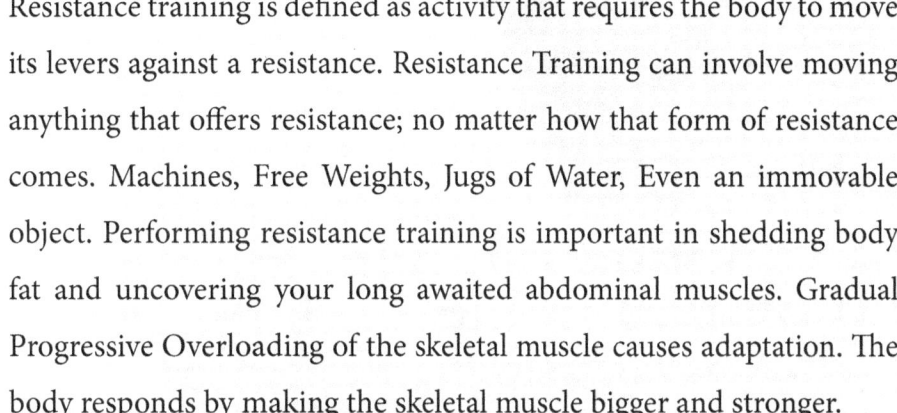

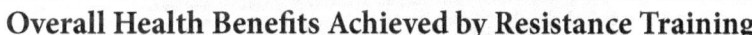

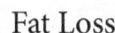

Overall Health Benefits Achieved by Resistance Training	
Fat Loss	Improved Strength / Functionability of Tendons & Tendons
Weight Maintenance	
Increased Calorie Expenditure during Rest and during Resistance Training	Increased Physical Independence
	Improved Posture
Reduction Blood Pressure	Improved Self – Esteem
Decreased Risk for Type II Diabetes	Improved Physical Image
Decreased Risk for Osteoporosis	
Increased Bone Mineral Content	

As previously mentioned, skeletal muscle is comprised of contractile pro-teins: Actin, Myosin, Troponin, and Tropomyosin. These contractile proteins grow largerthrough resistance training, rest and proper nutrition immediately following.

Before starting any resistance training program you should consult your physician to determine if you have any medical or health condition that would be cause for concern. Upon starting a resistance training program you should notice a difference in approximately 4-6 weeks, aligned within a sensible nutrition program (like the recommendations in Chapter 3) and rest.

Your body will specifically adapt to resistance training. Some of the changes will be visible to you in the mirror, some changes you will notice when engaging in a sporting event and some happen at the cellular or biologic level which is not as easily seen, but will garner health benefits for decades to come. Below is a partial list of just some of the adaptations you will undergo due

Variable	Results following Resistance Training
MUSCLE STRENGTH	INCREASES
MUSCLE ENDURANCE	INCREASES FOR HIGH POWER OUTPUT
MAX RATE OF FORCE PRODUCTION	INCREASES
VERTICAL JUMP	INCREASES
ANAEROBIC POWER	INCREASES
SPRINT SPEED	IMPROVES
FIBER SIZE	INCREASES
MITOCHONDRIAL DENSITY	DECREASES
FAST HEAVY CHAIN MYOSIN	INCREASES IN AMOUNT
ENZYME ACTIVITY	INCREASES FOR ENZYMES RELATED TO HIGH INTENSITY ACTIVITIES
STOERD ATP	INCREASES
STORED CREATINE PHOPHATE	INCREASES
STORED GLYCOGEN	INCREASES
FAT FREE MASS	**INCREASES**

Resistance training is a vital component to winning the war on fat, due in large part to a muscle's energy demand. For each pound of muscle you attain, the body burns approximately 15 additional calories per day at rest. Yes, that's right, the more muscle the more calories your body uses just to maintain that muscle.

Resistance training should not be solely relied on as a calorie burner. For a reduction in body fat and for obtaining your calorie deficit you should depend predominantly on cardiovascular exercise and nutrition. Resistance training uses sugar as fuel and is an anaerobic exercise. Resistance training should be used for stimulating muscle growth (hypertrophy). The key is to understand and acknowledge what types of exercises are needed and how often the repetition and weight.

The majority of traditional resistance training is referred to as isotonic training. "Iso" means "the same" and "tonic" means "tone or tension". That 20 pound dumbbell is always 20 pounds, from the beginning to the end of the exercise. In addition to Isotonic exercises there are also isometric exercises. "Iso" meaning "the same" and "metric" meaning length. The muscle contracts, but doesn't change lengths. Remember the old Charles Atlas advertisements in the back of comic books with the guy getting sand kicked in his face? Charles Atlas promoted isometric training. He would suggest pressing against an immovable object for strength. The only problem with training of this type is that strength develops only in that exact range of motion and angle (see S.A.I.D. Principle). The third type of contraction is the isokinetic contraction, "Iso" meaning "same" and "kinetic" meaning "speed or movement." This type of training requires costly machines and is usually performed as part rehabilitation therapy for an injury.

When you perform isotonic training, you are going to utilize a 6 second repetition. Within this six second interval is included four seconds of lowering the weight while inhaling or the eccentric portion of the exercise, and two seconds of raising the weight while exhaling also known as the concentric portion of the exercise.

(Note: Use of Valsalva's Maneuver, or holding one's breathing during the concentric portion of the lift, can lead to high blood pressure, ruptured alveoli and increased intra-occular pressure and is not promoted by this writer). Always exhale on the concentric portion of the lift.

To add lean body tissue when lifting, you want to maximize the amount of muscle used during your resistance training sessions. The more overall muscle applied to the exercise the more muscle you build. **Compound Exercises** are exercises that include movements at more than one joint and **Isolation Exercises** are exercises at only one joint. A flat bench barbell press is an example of a compound exercise for chest. The movement occurs at the elbow joint and the shoulder joint. A flat bench dumbbell fly is an example of an isolation exercise for the chest. The movement occurs only at the shoulder joint. Whereas, in the barbell flat bench press you stimulate the pectoralis major, anterior deltoid and triceps brachii muscles, in the flat bench dumbbell fly you predominantly use the pectoralis major muscle group with a little assistance from some of the stabilizer muscles of your core.

In order to achieve ultimate success in obtaining your new cheese grater stomach, you need to constantly push your body to adapt. One way to achieve employing this through resistance training is to use multiple training systems. The chart below describes training systems that will achieve this.

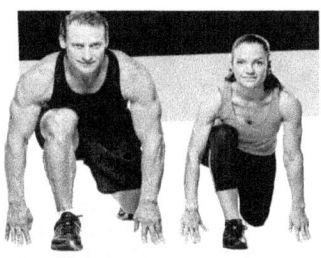

System	How to Perform	Benefits
Single Set	One set for each exercise	Good for beginners / General Health
Multiple Sets	Several sets of each exercise	General Fitness / Strength development
Super Set	Set of exercise A immediately followed by set of exercise B for opposing muscle group	Effective use of time, good for muscle hypertrophy
Tri Set	Several sets of three different exercises for the same Bodypart	Good for strength and muscle hypertrophy
Quad Set	Four sets of four different exercises for the same Bodypart	Good for strength and muscle hypertrophy
Light to Heavy	Progress from a light weight to heavier weight	Good for muscle endurance
Heavy to Light	Start with a Heavier Resistance and drop to lighter weights in subsequent sets	Good for Strength Gains
Pyramid Training	Light to Heavy Resistance then back to Light	Muscle hypertrophy and Muscle Endurance
Inverted Pyramid Training	Heavy to Light Resistance then back to Heavy	Muscle hypertrophy and Muscle Endurance, Benefit of more sets with heavier resistance
Drop Set / Strip Sets	Perform weight to failure or near failure , lower weight and proceed to failure again	Muscle hypertrophy and Muscle Endurance
Negative Training	Perform exercise to failure in concentric phase then perform slow eccentric repetitions while receiving assistance in concentric phases	Muscle Strength / Muscle Hypertrophy Gains / Leads to DOMS
Assisted Repetitions	Spotter assists in lifting of weight	Muscle Strength / Muscle Hypertrophy Gains
Compound Sets	Performing one set of an exercise immediately followed by a set of a different exercise for the same Bodypart	Muscle Strength / Muscle Hypertrophy Gains

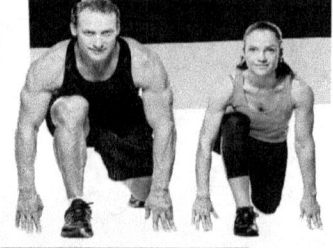

Rest Pause Sets	Performing repetitions with near maximal resistance, with rest periods in between repetitions	Increased Strength Gains
Super Slow Repetitions	Performing Repetitions in the 10-15 second range	Increased muscle endurance by increasing muscle's Time Under Tension (T.U.T.)
Blast Training	Performing Repetitions with near maximal speed in concentric phase while still using good form and maintaining normal eccentric timing	Good for Increased Strength / Power by recruiting more overall muscle fibers

Now that we've examined the different training systems that you will use during the next 12 weeks, lets take a look at the Major Body Parts and Compound Exercises that effectively target those muscles.

Bodypart	Exercise	Equipment Needed	Primary Muscle(s)	Secondary Muscle
Back	Pull-Ups	Pull Up Bar	Latissmus Dorsi, Posterior Deltoid, Teres Minor, Teres Major	Biceps Brachii, Brachialis, Brachioradialis
Back	Lat-Pull Down	Overhead Cable Machine	Latissmus Dorsi, Posterior Deltoid, Teres Minor, Teres Major	Biceps Brachii, Brachialis, Brachioradialis
Back	Bent Over Row	Barbell	Latissmus Dorsi, Poster Deltoid,	Teres Major, Teres Minor, Biceps Brachii, Brachialis
Back	Deadlifts	Barbell / Dumbbell	Traps I, II, III Erector Spinae	Hamstrings, Gluteus Maximus

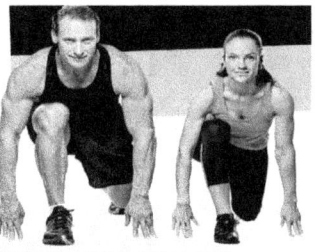

Back	T Bar Rows	T Bar Row Machine	Latissmus Dorsi	Biceps Brachii, Brachioradialis, Brachialis
Back	Seated Cable Row	Seated low cable pulley	Latissmus Dorsi, Teres Major, Posterior, Deltoids, Rhomboids, Trapezius	Biceps Brachii, Brachioradialis, BRachialis
Back	One Arm Dumbbell Row	Dumbbell	Latissmus Dorsi, Teres Major, Rhomboids, Trapezius	Biceps Brachii, Brachioradialis, BRachialis
Shoulders	Seated / Standing Barbell Press	Barbell	Anterior, Medial Deltoids, Upper Pectorals, Trapezius I	Triceps, Serratus Anterior
Shoulders	Seated / Standing Dumbbell Press	Dumbbell	Anterior, Medial Deltoids, Upper Pectorals, Trapezius I	Triceps, Serratus Anterior
Shoulders	Wide Barbell Upright Rows	Barbell	Medial Deltoids, Trapezius I	Brachioradialis, Brachialis
Chest Predominantly Mid to Lower	Flat Bench Press Barbell	Barbell, Bench	Pectoralis Major	Pectoralis Minor, Anterior Deltoid, Triceps Brachii
Chest Predominantly Mid to Lower	Flat Bench Press Dumbbell	Dumbbells, Flat Bench	Pectoralis Major	Pectoralis Minor, Anterior Deltoid, Triceps Brachii
Chest Predominantly Upper 1/3	Incline Bench Press Barbell	Barbell, Incline Bench (30° Incline)	Pectoralis Major	Pectoralis Minor, Anterior Deltoid, Triceps Brachii
Chest Predominantly Upper 1/3	Incline Bench Press Dumbbell	Dumbbell, Incline Bench (30°)	Pectoralis Major	Pectoralis Minor, Anterior Deltoid, Triceps Brachii

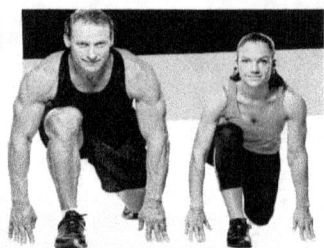

Chest Predominantly Mid to Lower 1/3	Decline Bench Press Barbell	Barbell, Decline Bench	Pectoralis Major	Pectoralis Minor, Anterior Deltoid, Triceps Brachii
Chest Predominantly Mid to Lower 1/3	Decline Bench Press Dumbbell	Dumbbells, Decline Bench	Pectoralis Major	Pectoralis Minor, Anterior Deltoid, Triceps Brachii
Chest Predominantly Mid to Lower 1/3	Dips	Parallel Dip Bars	Pectoralis Major	Pectoralis Minor, Anterior Deltoid, Triceps Brachii
Legs	Barbell Squat	Barbell, Squat Rack	Vastus Medialis, Vastus Lateralis, Vastus Intermedius, Rectus Femoris, and Gluteus Maximus	Gastrocnemius, Soleus, Rectus Abdominis, Erector Spinae
Legs	Dumbbell Squat	Dumbbells	Vastus Medialis, Vastus Lateralis, Vastus Intermedius, Rectus Femoris, and Gluteus Maximus Intermedius and Rectus Femoris, Gluteus Maximus	Gastrocnemius, Soleus, Rectus Abdominis, Erector Spinae
Legs	Smith Machine Squat	Smith Machine	Vastus Medialis, Vastus Lateralis, Vastus Intermedius, Rectus Femoris, and Gluteus Maximus	Gastrocnemius, Soleus, Rectus Abdominis, Erector Spinae

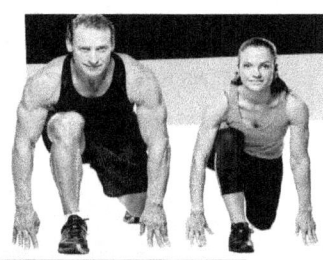

Legs	Leg Press	Leg Press Machine	Vastus Medialis, Vastus Lateralis, Vastus Intermedius, Rectus Femoris, and Gluteus Maximus *(Foot planted lower on Plate)	
Legs	Leg Press	Leg Press Machine	Gluteus Maximus, Hamstring Group	
Traps	Barbell Shrugs	Barbell	Trapezius I, II, Medial, Posterior Deltoids	Forearm Flexors
Traps	Dumbbell Shrugs	Dumbbells	Trapezius I, II, Medial, Posterior Deltoids	Forearm Flexors
Traps	Close Grip Upright Rows	Barbell	Trapezius I, II, Medial, Posterior Deltoids	Forearm Flexors, Brachioradialis, Brachialis
Biceps	Underhand Close Grip Pull-Ups	Pull Up Bar	Biceps Brachii, Brachialis, Brachioradialis	Latissimus Dorsi, Teres Major, Posterior Deltoids
Biceps	Straight / EZ Bar Curls	Straight Bar, EZ Bar	Biceps Brachii, Brachialis, Brachioradialis	Pronator Teres, Forearm Flexors
Biceps	Seated / Standing Dumbbell Curls	Dumbbells	Biceps Brachii, Brachialis, Brachioradialis	Pronator Teres, Forearm Flexors
Triceps	Dips (Elbows in tight)	Parallel Dip Bars	Triceps Brachii	Pectoralis Major, Anterior Deltoid

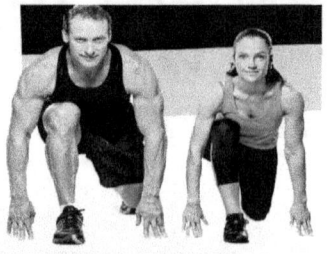

Triceps	Close Grip Barbell Bench Press	Barbell, Flat Bench	Triceps Brachii	Pectoralis Major, Anterior Deltoid
Triceps	Overhead Dumbbell Extensions	Dumbbell	Triceps Brachii (long head, Lateral Head)	
Calves*	Standing Barbell Raises	Barbell	Gastrocnemius	Soleus
Calves*	Seated Calf Raises (Machine)	Seated Calf Raise Machine	Soleus	Gastrocnemius
Calves*	Standing Dumbbell Calf Raises	Dumbbells	Gastrocnemius	Soleus

* If legs are straight 90% of work is done by Gastrocnemius (commonly referred to as the calf), if legs are bent 90% of work is performed by Soleus (or the deep calf muscle).

For the first 12 week session, you will not employ advanced techniques or training systems. Refer back to the chart if you are unsure of what are considered advanced.

Below you will find a sample week of resistance training. You will choose one exercise per body part working the entire body each session (a description of each exercise can be found in the appendix). Each exercise will be performed in three sets of 8-12 repetitions per set. The resistance used should cause failure or near failure within the prescribed repetition range. A rest period between each set should be kept at 60 seconds or until breathing and heart rate has returned to normal. The exercises that are being shown are compound in nature. Remember compound exercises use overall more muscles and thus produce greater gains than isolation exercises.

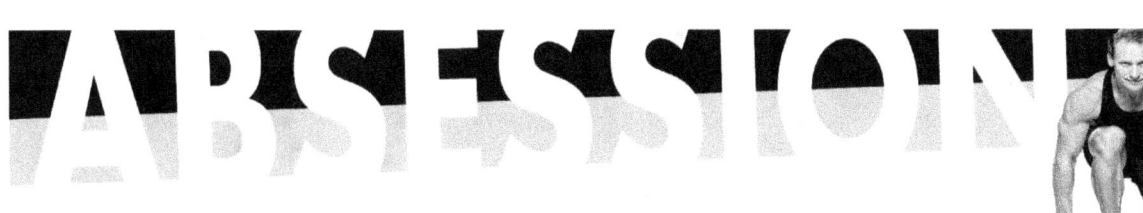

ABSESSION

In the model below, the 3 days of resistance training has been set up as a Monday, Wednesday, Friday routine. However, you may change that to any convenient schedule as long as one day falls in between.

SAMPLE WEEK"S RESISTANCE TRAINING

MONDAY	WEDNESDAY	FRIDAY
Chest Flat Bench Barbell	**Chest** Incline Dumbbell Press	**Chest** Decline Barbell Press
Back Pull-ups	**Back** Bent Over Barbell Rows	**Back** T Bar Rows
Shoulders Seated Dumbbell Press	**Shoulders** Standing Barbell Press	**Shoulders** Upright Barbell Rows (wide)
Legs Dumbbell Squats	**Legs** Barbell Squats	**Legs** Leg Press
Biceps Straight Bar Curl	**Biceps** Seated Dumbbell Curls	**Biceps** Underhand Close Grip Pull-ups
Triceps Dips	**Triceps** Close Grip Barbell Bench Press	**Triceps** Overhead Dumbbell Extensions
Calves Standing Barbell Calf Raises	**Calves** Seated Calf Raises	**Calves** Standing Dumbbell Calf Raises

The above chart of resistance training is just an example of how to put together a week of exercise sessions. You can go to the major muscle parts and exercises chart to choose any one exercise for any Bodypart and design your own. Use the Weight Training Chart located in the Forms Section to record weight used and repetitions so you can track your improvements.

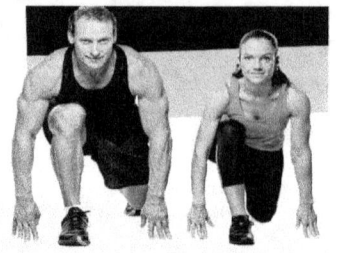
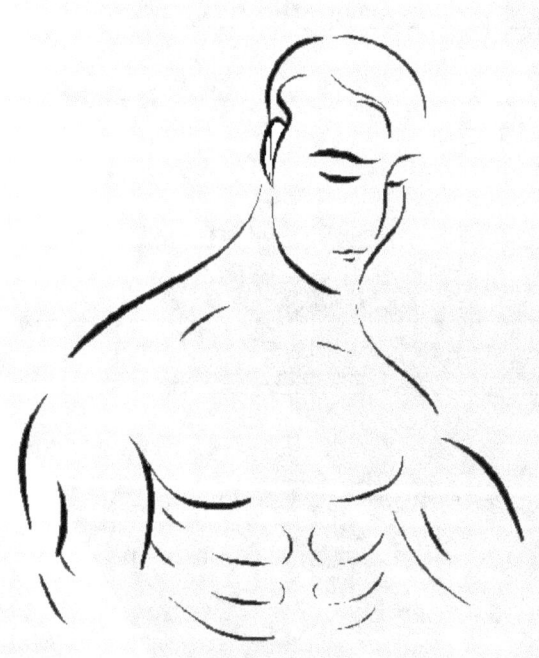

ABSESSION

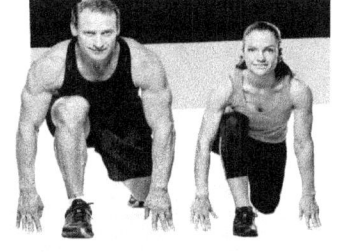

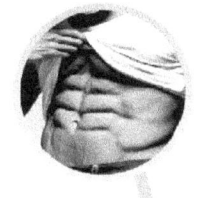

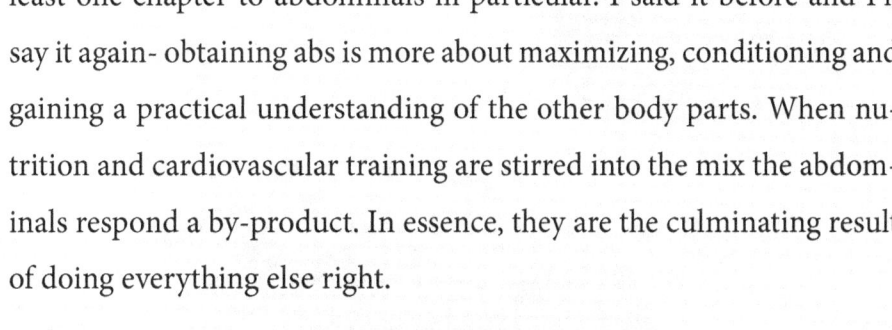

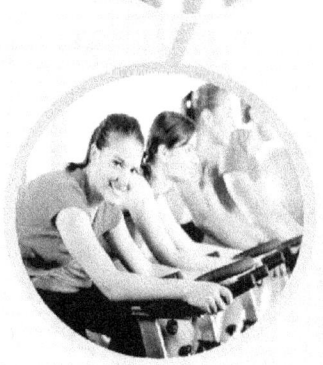

I guess I couldn't really call this book "Absession" if I didn't devote at least one chapter to abdominals in particular. I said it before and I'll say it again- obtaining abs is more about maximizing, conditioning and gaining a practical understanding of the other body parts. When nutrition and cardiovascular training are stirred into the mix the abdominals respond a by-product. In essence, they are the culminating result of doing everything else right.

Where do people's eyes go to when they see someone? Ask yourself, "after the initial pleasantries, and eye to eye contact, where do you look?" The center, the core, the middle the mid section etc! Whatever you want to call it – the abdominal region, pulls it all together. A firm, lean stomach makes the chest more pronounced, the shoulders wider, the back broader and the legs more flared. It is the center of it all - the crossroads of a perfect "X shape". Unfortunately, too many Americans are a few letters off in the alphabet- they resemble more a "U shape" (U for underachiever) or a side shot "D shape" (D for disgusting) – anyway, you get the point.

Look at Greek Statues, what is the most pronounced body part on Michelangelo's David- One guess, it's not his distended gut. Rather, it is a

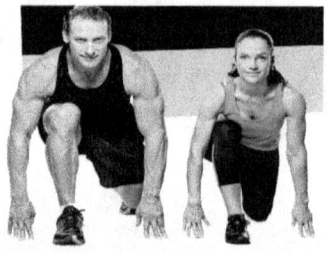

other body parts. A firm mid section is pleasing to the eyes, shows self control, power and determination.

A set of well defined abdominals and a loss of upper torso body fat are not only important for aesthetic reasons. In addition, it's a major health concern. Upper body fat increases a person's risk for type II Diabetes, and heart disease, not to mention that the majority of low back pain can be attributed to both weak abdominals and an overabundance of upper body fat.

The key to a fine set of deeply etched abdominals is 90% nutrition. I know I'll see raised eyebrows and hear vocal opposition, but I'd venture to say only the remaining 10% is comprised of cardio and resistance training. Did you notice I didn't say anything about direct abdominal exercises? You can crunch, do sit ups, and perform leg lifts from forever, yet with 20 extra pounds of fat hanging over your belt; your hard work will be anticlimactic. You will never see the fruits of your labor hidden beneath mounds of fat. You will be healthier yes, but overweight.

I know this is not an epiphany - **"Spot Reduction is Impossible"** – I've said it before in this book and yet I say it again – Why? Because all one needs to do is turn on any late night infomercial and you'll see endless ab-gizmos being hawked. TV time is not free, so someone must be buying these worthless contraptions. Just to paraphrase our earlier chapter, your body uses fat holistically from your body. This means you are either in a fat burning mode or you are not. You can not dial up your love handles exclusively and use that fat for energy. It just doesn't work that way!!

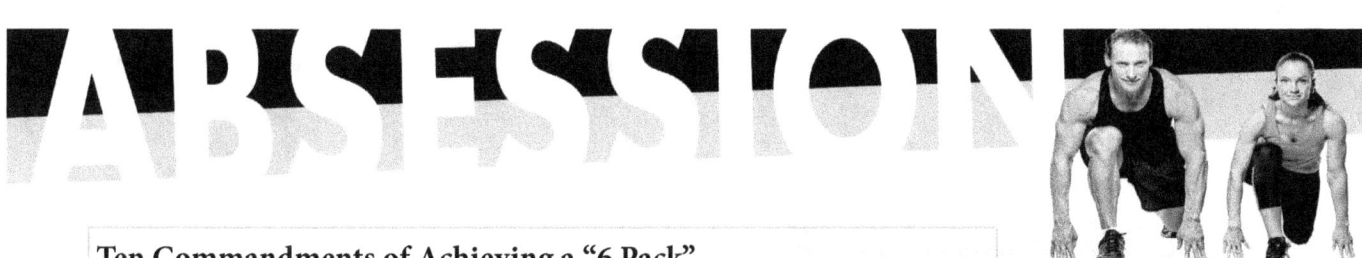

Ten Commandments of Achieving a "6 Pack"

1. Reduce Your Body Fat

- You could possess the most sharply defined set of abs known to man, but whether covered by a thin sheath or bulky covering of fat, no one will ever see them. Remember body fat levels are held in check by proper nutrition and cardiovascular exercise.

2. The Rectus Abdominis is one muscle, with one origin and one insertion.

- The Rectus Abdominis has an origin of the pubic bone and an insertion point of the sternum (xiphoid process). You can not target upper or lower abs.

3. If your xiphoid process and your umbilicus do not move closer to one another, you

- In order to stimulate the Rectus Abdominis, the xiphoid process and the umbilicus must move closer to each other. The Rectus Abdominis' main functions to flex the trunk and provide lower back stabilization.

4. Your abdominals get plenty of peripheral work each and every day.

- Believe it or not, your abdominal region experiences sufficient stimulation (albeit a lot of isometric contraction), by maintaining good posture throughout the day. The transverse Abdominis (your deep abdominal muscle) helps maintain good posture and is also activated throughout the day and through cardiovascular exercise.

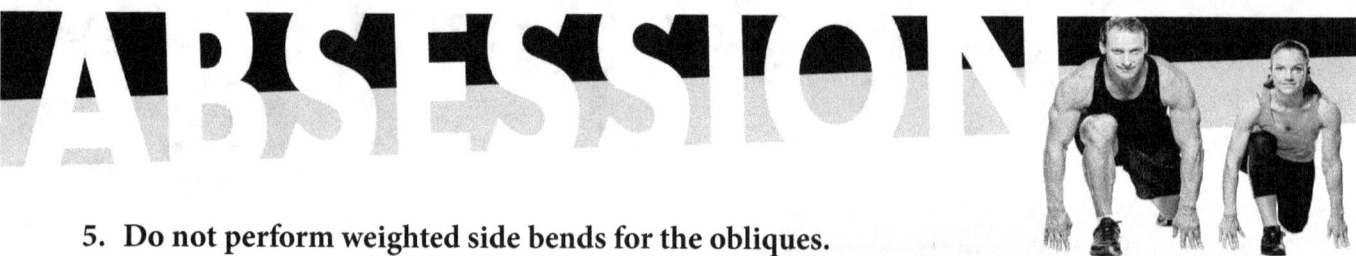

5. Do not perform weighted side bends for the obliques.

- Weighted side bends are not advisable for two reasons: 1) they place the spine in a susceptible position for injury while under load and 2) when worked they bring about hypertrophy (growth) for the obliques causing the waist to appear big and blocky.

6. Do not perform ab exercises each day.

- Your abdominal region is comprised of muscles. Much like chest, back or shoulders, muscles grow and get stronger after they are stimulated through resistance training, but more so in conjunction with proper rest and nutritional intake.

7. You can't crunch away your fat.

- You can not spot reduce.

8. Learn the benefit of isometric contractions

- Performing the plank, or just contracting your abs throughout the day while at work, play or driving, will bring about a stronger core and even some muscular endurance in the abdominal region.

9. Do not forget to train spinal erectors.

- Any good training program promotes muscle symmetry. Neglecting to train the spinal erectors will only hamper your development and can lead to muscle imbalance and lead to injury.

10. Avoid straight leg sit ups

- Straight leg sit ups place the lower back at risk by placing a large amount of stress on it. In addition, the hip flexors are engaged, thus diverting the required tension away from the abdominals.

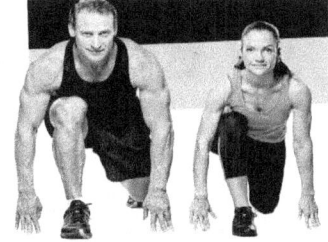
Specific Abdominal Exercises

Rope handle Crunches

Primary muscle: Rectus Abdominis.

Synergistic muscle(s): Serratus anterior, Intercostals.

- Begin with rope attached to overhead pulley.

- While facing away from machine grasp handles behind head while kneeling approximately

   a foot away from machine.

- Bend forward at waist until Rectus Abdominis is fully contracted.

- Exhale as abdominals contract.

- Continue for desired number of repetitions.

- Concentric portion of exercise should take two seconds.

- Exhale during concentric portion.

- Eccentric portion of the exercise should take four seconds.

- Inhale during eccentric portion.

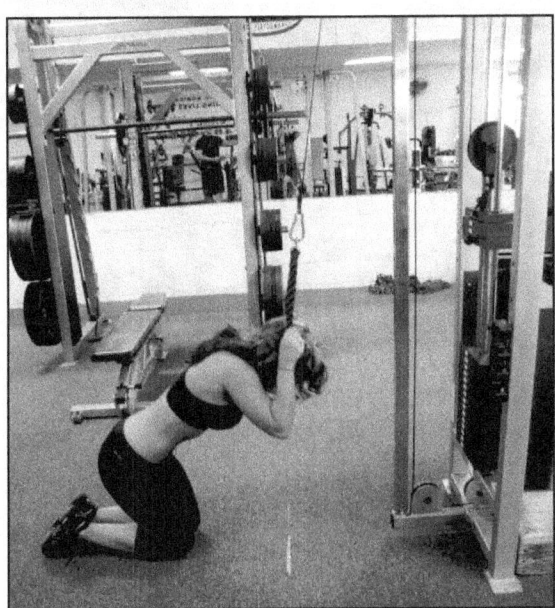
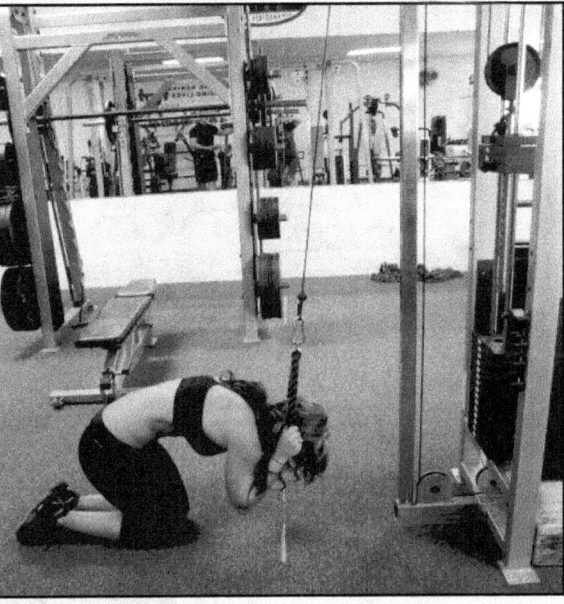

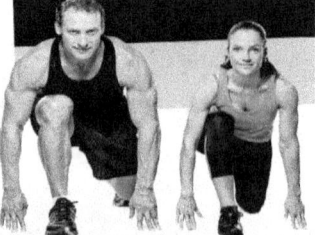

Knee ups

Primary muscle: Rectus Abdominis

Synergistic muscle(s): Hip flexors, Illiopsoas

- Begin by sitting on the end of a flat bench.

- Place hands behind hips on bench for support.

- Start with legs extended.

- Pull knees to chest area.

- Contract abdominals and exhale.

- Continue for desired number of repetitions.

- Concentric portion of the lift should take two seconds.

- Eccentric portion of the lift should take four seconds

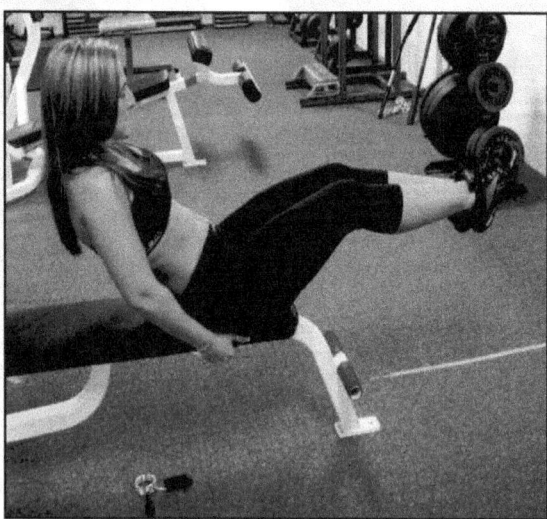
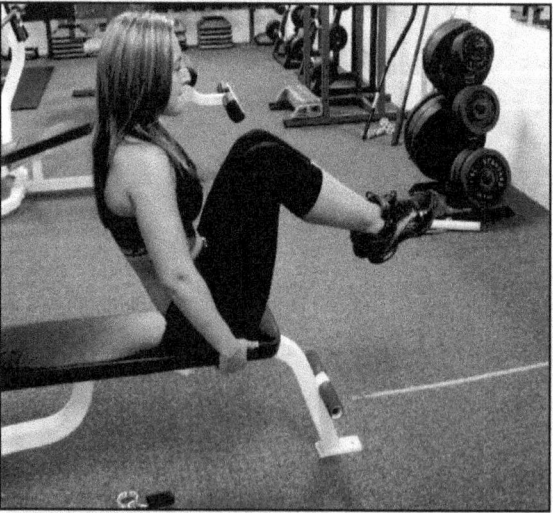

Crunches

Primary muscle(s): Rectus Abdominis

- Begin by lying flat of the floor or decline bench with knees bent (a swiss ball can also be used).

- Place hands across chest or under chin (to avoid pulling on neck).

- Raise upper torso by contacting abdominals.

- Exhale as upper body raises.

- Slowly descend, do not return all the way to making contact with either the floor or bench (this will remove tension from the abdominals).

- Continue for desired number of repetitions.

- Concentric portion of the exercise should take two seconds.

- Eccentric portion of the exercise should take four seconds.

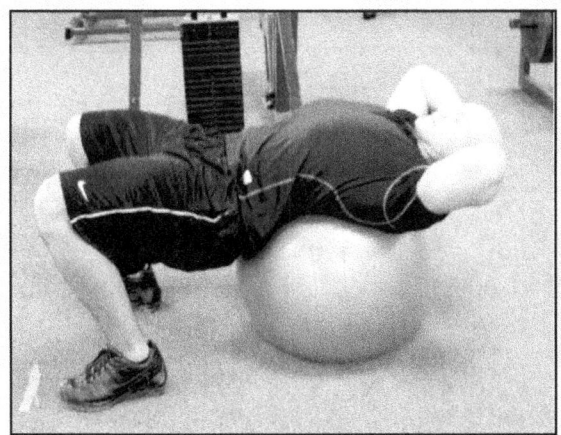 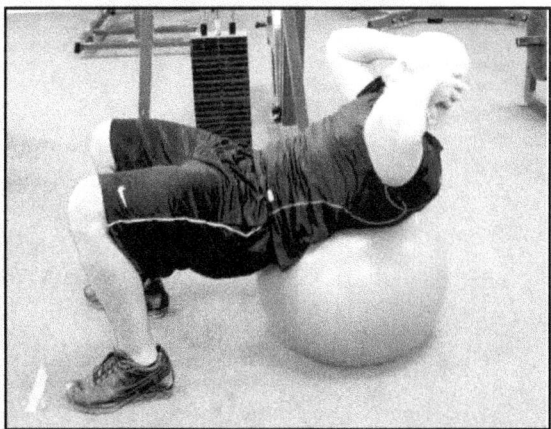

Roman Chair Knee Raises

Primary muscle(s): Rectus Abdominis

Synergistic muscle(s): Serratus Anterior, Hip Flexors, Illiopsoas

- Being by supporting body weight on arms

- Start with legs straight down in hanging position

- Slowly contract abdominals while lifting knees upward

- Roll hips at top of movement, thus shortening the distance between zyphoid process and umbilicus

- Return to starting position

- Repeat for desired number of repetitions

- Concentric portion of the exercise should take two seconds

- Eccentric portion of the exercise should take four seconds

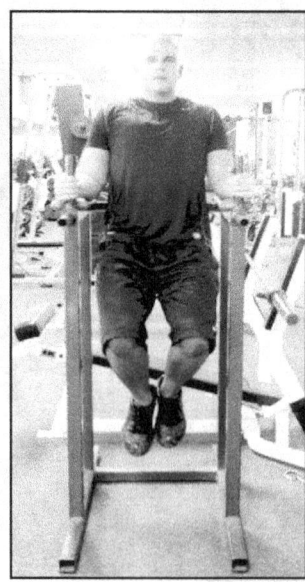 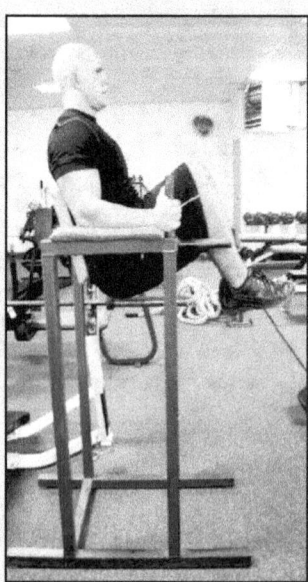

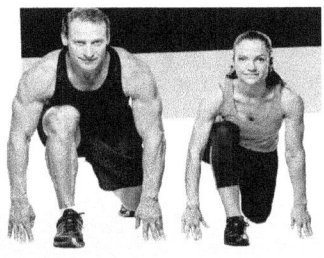

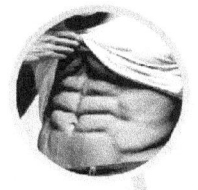

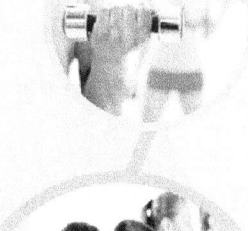

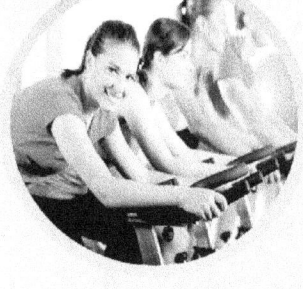

Well , we have explored Cardiovascul ar / Aerobic Training, Resistance Training, and Nutrition. We have examined the energy systems and the process of muscular contraction. We have also touched on how macronutrients are metabol ized, used for fuel and **utilized to either build muscle or body fat**. Ok, that's itbest of luck to you! Just ki dding, I wouldn't do that we now have reached another important issue that can make or break your decision to look fit and be fit. We must pull it all together.

What I strongly suggest you do is commit one hour a day to this program – one hour that's it! Do it and you will have the body you have always wanted. Give yourself 12 weeks, follow the program and you wi ll realize a leaner body, a more toned body, with a mid section that is all but non-existent.

Remember everything we covered about cardiovascular exercise and proper exerci se intensities. Remember to use our compound, multi joint resistance exercises 3 days a week. Remember especial ly, to watch your nutrition and make wi se food choices. It matters most what you put into your body for fuel when training. Don't sabotage great cardi o and weight workouts by eating garbage. The old computer saying fits in nicely here-GARBAGE IN = GARBAGE OUT!!! If you put garbage in your body, your body wil l reflect garbage on the outside.

This brings us finally to the topic heading – visualization. If you have never attempted visualization exercises let me introduce you to one, simple example. I would like you to visualize your new body. Visualize a fit, trim, healthier you. Hold that image and recall the minimal effort you exerted and the better food choices you opted for in order to reach that goal. The key phrases here are "minimal effort" and "better food choices."

With that visualization in mind, picture yourself going somewhere, anywhere, where your friends knew the "old you." Their previous mental image of you will obviously differ from your visualization. One final step; Make that visualization a reality. How great would you feel when those same friends comment of your improvements, ask how you accomplished that goal, admire the willpower it demonstrates.

I have always operated under the premise that if you can believe it, you can achieve it. What makes a world class athlete, a better athlete? Were they simply blessed with superior genetics? Maybe, but not solely! They visualize. They see themselves being successful at their chosen sport long before the event ever takes place. They see themselves again and again, hitting the game winning shot at the buzzer, throwing the last second touchdown pass, hitting the winning homerun in the bottom of the ninth with two outs. It is in the mind's eye so much can make good on it.

Before something manifests itself externally, it must be clearly defined and visualized internally. In other words, you can't get somewhere; if you don't know where you want to go. This technique will definitely work for you. Visualize toned and muscular and you will achieve it. Visualization is the germ of that achievement. Visualize yourself to better health. Eventually, your body will follow and you will become what you have always wanted to be.

You obviously have the picture. Now, with your focus of attention on your goal add three more visualizations.

- Imagine you have skipped a workout.

- Imagine that your workout effort is lackluster or half hearted.

- Imagine making poor nutrition choices.

A question arises, and the question is this.......
"Who are you cheating?"

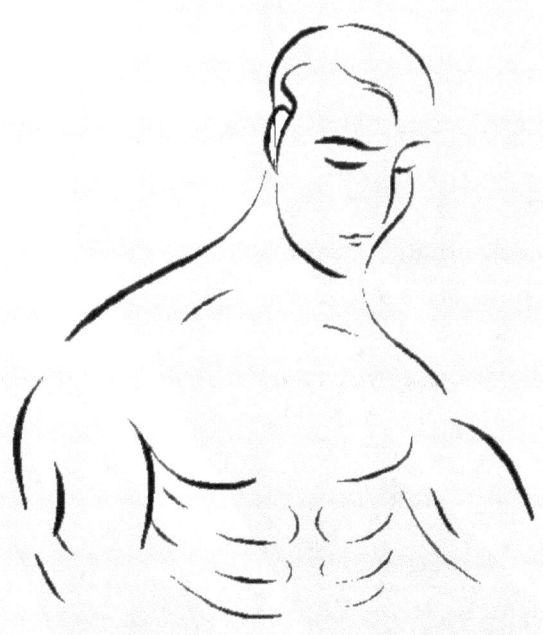

"Winning starts with beginning" -
Anonymous

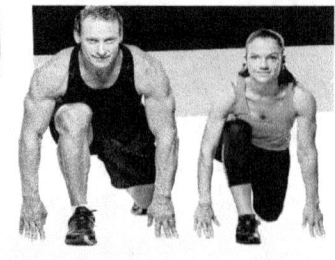

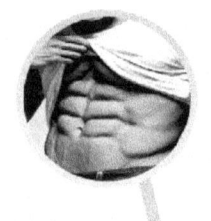

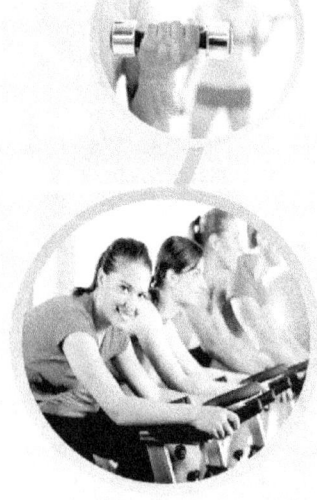

Q. Can I selectively lose fat just off my abs and keep size every where else?

A. *According to current research, the body uses stored fat for energy holistically; you cannot target one bodypart.*

Q. I've seen those rubber belts with Velcro for your midsection, do they work?

A. *Waist trimmers will make you thinner in only one place, your wallet. You cannot spot reduce!!!*

Q. I've heard that light weight and high repetitions will "cut me up" and help my abs show through- is this true?

A. *Muscle is metabolically active so building more muscle burns more calories. It is accomplished by the gradual progression of resistance to overload the muscle. Hitting failure or near failure between 8-12 repetitions will maximize this process.*

Q. My friend says walking is just as effective at burning fat as jogging – is he correct?

A. *If you have no medical condition that prohibits you from jogging, then jogging is more effective. If it takes you an hour to walk 4 miles as opposed to jogging four miles in 40 minutes (ten minute miles), you have done the same amount in distance, but you have performed more overall work, thus burning more calories. More work performed, more calories used.*

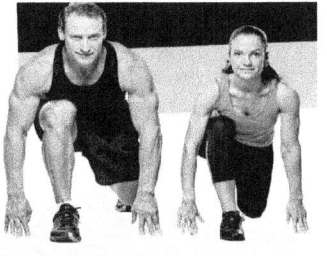

Q. What is better for burning fat- low intensity or higher intensity aerobic activity?

A. *Low intensity uses a greater % of fat calories than high intensity; however the overall number of calories is smaller. Thus fewer fat calories are used for energy. A combination of low intensity, longer duration sessions coupled with sessions of higher intensities gives you the best of both worlds for your attack on fat. Go back and read Chapter 2.*

Q. I read once that if you perform weighted Abdominal exercises, it will build muscle and the added muscle will "pop" the abs through the fat- is this true?

A. *Attaining the visible 6 pack is a product of low body fat. Attained by a combination of cardiovascular exercise and a sound nutritional program. If you build up your abdominal muscles by resistance training and still hold 20% bodyfat you just won't see them.*

Q. Should I perform weighted abdominal exercises?

A. *A strong core is very important for functional fitness. There is nothing wrong with performing some weighted Ab exercises along with lower back exercises to strengthen your core. I would stay away from direct weighted oblique exercises. The obliques respond like other skeletal muscle, by growing larger in size to resistance training. Thicker obliques lead to a thicker waistline.*

Q. I've heard that the only way to "target" the lower abs is through leg lifts- is this true?

A. *The Rectus Abdominis is one muscle with one origin and one insertion. You cannot effectively target or isolate the lower abs. Dialing in the bottom part of the Rectus Abdominis is more a result of low bodyfat, achieved by cardiovascular exercise and a diligent nutrition plan.*

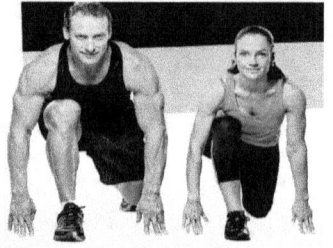

Q. My friend suggested I eat a candy bar prior to working out for "quick energy", how will this effect my weight training session?

A. *First off, you want to minimize simple carbohydrates from your diet. Remember simple carbohydrates will be converted to stored bodyfat more readily than complex carbohydrates. Secondly, prior to resistance training it is more advisable to eat a slow digesting carbohydrate with a protein source to maintain adequate energy levels throughout your workout. You definitely do not want to experience a rapid rise and drop in blood sugar while resistance training. Immediately following your workout would be the only time I would suggest consuming a faster digesting carbohydrate with a protein source. This will take advantage of the body's natural occurring hormone insulin. Insulin will move the nutrients (glucose and amino acids) out of the blood and into the muscle cell receptor sites, ultimately moving you out of a state of catabolism and into a state of anabolism. With this being said, I still believe there are better food choices (even post workout) than a candy bar.*

Q. If 3500 kcals equal one pound of fat, why can't I just go on a calorie restricted diet of 500-1000 calories a day and lose weight?

A. *The problem with this scenario is as follows: the body is much too efficient to be "tricked" like this. What your body attempts to do when it recognizes such a dramatic reduction in calories is sacrifice lean muscle tissue, and in extreme cases even organ tissue, to manufacture the calories need to survive. In addition, once you return to a more normal caloric intake regiment, the body is now a less efficient "fat burner" because you now possess less muscle.*

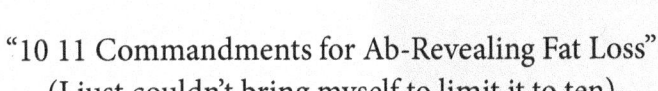

"10 11 Commandments for Ab-Revealing Fat Loss"
(I just couldn't bring myself to limit it to ten)

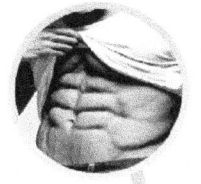

This is the point I will attempt to summarize Fat Loss. A revelation which ultimately is your guide to abtaining (oops sorry), obtaining your six pack. I could have started with this disclosure on page one but two major purposes would not have been accomplished;

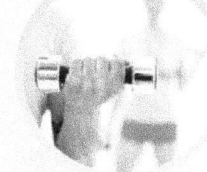

You would be following a so-called 12 week program, without understanding the Why's behind it. A learning gap would exist concerning Energy Systems, the Body's Response to Resistance Training, Nutrition and the Anatomy and Physiology of the Human Body. I am a firm believer in the age old parable; "Feed a man a fish and he eats for a meal, but teach a man to fish and he eats a lifetime". So consider this book as your Fishing 101 Guide for Life.

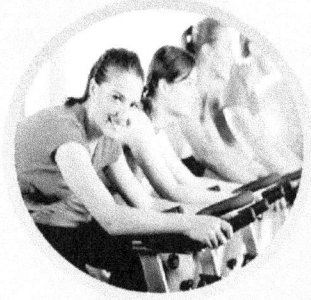

The second equally important omission is self-serving. I never would have been able to publish this book, assuming it only included this list.

All joking aside, it is critical to understand the why's, so if ever you fall off the wagon from your previous gluttonous state, you can catch yourself, reinstitute the program and forever be the "Master of Your Body." You will no longer be the victim of the "runaway train syndrome", in which you cannot stop repeating poor, detrimental habits.

A commandment is a precept that must be obeyed by those concerned. Are you concerned? If so, these tips are for you. Because all are important to the quest for your best, the following list is in no particular order.

1. Cardio for Fat Loss

Cardiovascular exercise is a must for fat loss. The key to maximize fat loss is somewhat of a shell game, keep your body guessing and ultimately adapting. Performing cardio at a mind numbing rate of ten minutes per mile for 1 hour is not going to result in the Abs of your dreams. Your body adapts very quickly and systematically using less energy in the form of fat to accomplish the same amount of work. By consistently changing the stimuli, your body has no other choice but to adapt and continue to use fat stores as fuel.

2. Document Everything

Become a stickler for documentation. If it goes in your mouth, document it, if you lift it, run it, peddle it – Write it Down!! Try it for just a day. You will not believe how much you actually ingest in 8 waking hours, but you just might hold yourself accountable if you document everything. In addition to recording food consumption benefits, document your workouts. It will prove to be an invaluable resource when training enabling you to push yourself harder and farther than you ever believed was possible.

3. Don't Eat by Accident – Have a Plan

"People don't plan to fail, they fail to plan." No comment could be more appropriate, when it comes to food choices. For the majority of people, you eat out of boredom or out of convenience; boredom because you failed to time and space out your meals accordingly, convenience because you are looking for that quick meal. You failed to plan and prepare food, so you go through a drive-through or you call up and order that pizza. Make a plan. Address both the boredom and convenience landmines that plague everyone that desires a better body.

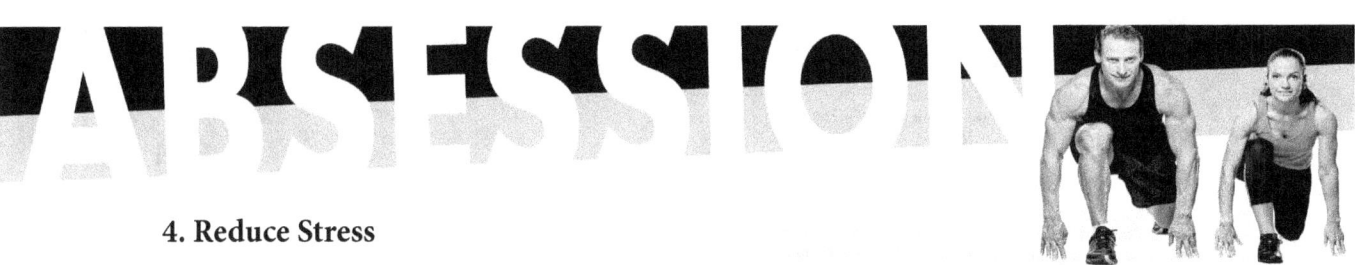

4. Reduce Stress

In addition to all of the noted health ailments that stress manifests, stress also releases the hormone cortisol, which reduces fat release and ultimately causes your body to hoard fat – a very undesirable state for anyone wishing to uncover his or her best body.

5. Reward Yourself

Remember, in order to continue on this path you cannot view it as a punishment. If necessary take one meal a week and enjoy your favorite food. You will benefit in two ways. First, the meal will represent a welcome change-of-pace for your spirit. Knowing you have not completely isolated yourself from your former life is reassuring. Second, it will give your body an increase in calories keeping your body in a fat burning mode, a little bonus. Remember you want your body to continue to adapt and you must give it a reason to do so.

6. Water, Water, Water

Water is the universal medium for all the body's metabolic functions. It also will give you a level of satiety. Unlike many other liquids such as coffee, tea or soda, water can create that full feeling. Natural diuretics, both coffee and tea contain caffeine which will dehydrate the body and take away from its ability to function at maximum capacity. The same is true for diet soda, while containing no sugar does contain artificial sweeteners, which have been shown in studies to actually increase hunger.

7. Don't miss or skip workouts (Embrace the fitness lifestyle as a way of life)

Performing the same activity for three consecutive days will make it a habit. Do not view these next twelve weeks of your life as simply a start date and an end date. In order to achieve unparalleled success compared with previous unsuccessful attempts, you must consider this a re-birth of sorts. This born again mentality will aid you in embracing the fitness lifestyle and ultimately help you achieve your best level of fitness ever!

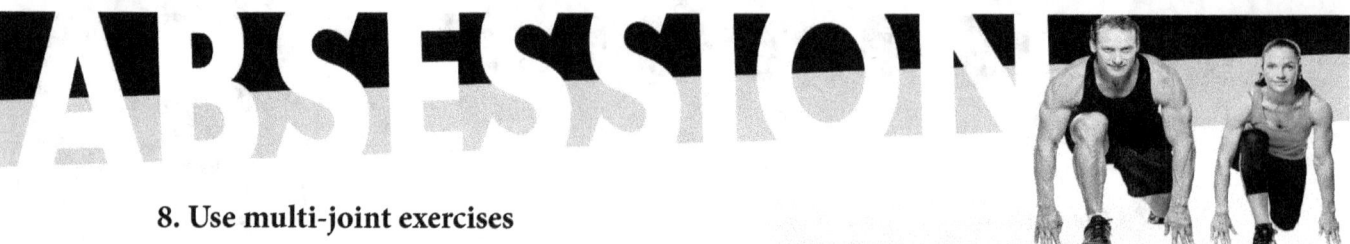

8. Use multi-joint exercises

Multi-joint exercises use more overall muscle, which in turn builds more overall muscle. Not only will this assist you in becoming more toned and lean, but you will also benefit from the increased calorie expenditure from the rise in lean muscle you now proudly carry on your body.

9. Weight training before Cardiovascular exercise, if both are being performed during the same exercise session

Resistance training uses glucose and stored glycogen as energy. Cardiovascular exercise, when performed correctly, uses Fat. If you perform your cardiovascular exercise after your resistance training you will tap into fat stores sooner because your glycogen stores fueled your resistance training.

10. Get more Rest

Inside a gym, everybody believes that they are marshaling energy, directing it, improving, growing. Actually, you make your greatest gains, after you work out. Proper nutrition and rest help. While sleeping the body releases growth hormones which enables your body to recuperate and return stronger, leaner and more vital. Remember, training places your body in a state of catabolism.

11. Visualize

Half the battle is in your mind – visualize your success. What the mind can conceive the body will achieve. The most important battle to win is the internal, personal battle in your mind. Don't think back to previous failed attempts at weight loss or long forgotten training programs. You will succeed this time; you will become that person you've always wanted to be. No longer will you dread buying clothes or looking in a mirror. Your poor body image is a thing of the past.

ABSESSION

Week	Sun	Mon	Tue	Wed	Thu	Fri	Sat
1	OFF	Resistance Training **Remember: Form is Key**	Cardio Training 15-20 Minutes Low Intensity	Resistance Training	Cardio Training 15-20 Minutes Low Intensity	Resistance Training	Cardio Training **Cheat Meal** 15-20 Minutes Low Intensity
2	OFF	Resistance Training **Concentrate on Breathing** **2 Seconds Concentric,** **4 Seconds Eccentric**	Cardio Training 20 25 Minutes Low Intensity	Resistance Training	Cardio Training 20-25 Minutes Low Intensity	Resistance Training	Cardio Training **Cheat Meal** 20-25 Minutes Low Intensity
3	OFF	Resistance Training **Increase Weight on Exercises if achieving 12 Repetitions**	Cardio Training Increase Time to 25-30 Minutes	Resistance Training **Remember Your Nutritional Recommendations**	Cardio Training Increase Time to 25-30 Minutes	Resistance Training	Cardio Training **Cheat Meal** Increase Time to 25-30 Minutes

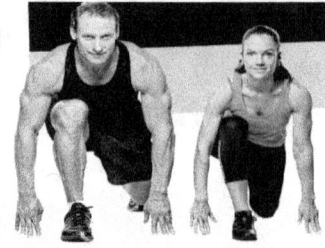

4	OFF	Resistance Training **Remember:** One pound of muscle burns up to 15 extra calories per day	Cardio Training 30-35 Minutes	Resistance Training	Cardio Training 25 minutes @ 75% MHR	Resistance Training	Cardio Training **Cheat Meal** 30-35 Minutes
5	OFF	Resistance Training	Cardio Training 20-25 Minutes / Alternating between 75-60% MHR	Resistance Training	Cardio Training 35-40 Minutes @ 60-70% MHR	Resistance Training	Cardio Training **Cheat Meal**
6	OFF	Resistance Training	Cardio Training 40-45 Minutes @ 60-70% MHR	Resistance Training Remember your water intake	Cardio Training	Resistance Training 40-45 Minutes @ 60-70% MHR	Cardio Training Cheat Meal 40-45 Minutes @ 60-70% MHR
7	OFF	Resistance Training Change Compound Exercises this Week for 2 Bodyparts	Cardio Training Increase Time to 25-30 Minutes	Resistance Training	Cardio Training 45-50 Minutes @ 60-70% MHR	Resistance Training	Cardio Training **Cheat Meal 25-30 Minutes Alternating Between 60-80% MHR**

8	OFF	Resistance Training	Cardio Training 30-35 Minutes Alternating between 80-65% MHR	Resistance Training	Cardio Training 50-55 Minutes @ 60-70% MHR	Resistance Training	Cardio Training 50-55 Minutes @ 60-70% MHR
9	OFF	Resistance Training	Cardio Training Change Mode of Cardio this Week.	Resistance Training	Cardio Training	Resistance Training	Cardio Training **Cheat Meal**
10	OFF	Resistance Training Remember your water	Cardio Training	Resistance Training	Cardio Training	Resistance Training	Cardio Training **Cheat Meal**
11	OFF	Resistance Training Change Compound Exercises this Week for 2 Bodyparts	Cardio Training	Resistance Training	Cardio Training	Resistance Training	Cardio Training **Cheat Mcal**
12	OFF	Resistance Training	Cardio Training	Resistance Training	Cardio Training	Resistance Training	Cardio Training **Cheat Meal**

The road to fitness is always under construction. It is a progressive, constantly evolving course. It is not a one-time destination. It is filled with many pitfalls. It is not easily navigated. With holidays, weddings, picnics and Super Bowl parties eminently tempting you with poor nutritional choices and missed workouts it isn't easy. This program is here to begin and continue your success. Now, you possess a definitive, clear-cut, holistic plan of attack. You now possess strategic knowledge of weights, workouts and timing to maximize fat loss. You now know how much food you need to lose fat and increase lean muscle. You also understand the body's true nutritional requirements, what to eat and when.

The only thing not discussed may well be the very thing holding you back. It may be the essence of your previous failed attempts at getting into great shape and developing a 6 pack that others envied. You may very well be lacking the *faith* that you **will** do it. Think about it. The defin-

much more appropriate can you get? Somewhere underneath all of the cheeseburgers, pizza, ice cream and sugar laden drinks exists a 6 pack.

There are two types of people; People who allow fitness to define their lives and people who allow it to enrich their lives. My hope for you is that you strive to be the latter of the two.

Today is the day "we" start to uncover the real you, the you that was meant to be, the you that intended on being all along.

Best of Luck and God Bless,

Scott

Glossary

Acetic Acid – the end product of the anaerobic breakdown of glucose

Acetyl CoA –An energy intermediate stimulated by eating above and beyond basal caloric needs. It is required in order to enter into the Krebs Cycle for energy production. (Also known as the "Gatekeeper".)

Actin – the thinner of the 2 contractile proteins that resides within the myofibril of the muscle.

Adenosine Di-Phosphate – is the resultant molecule when Adenosine Tri- Phosphate releases one of its phosphates for energy.

Adenosine Tri-Phosphate- is a high energy molecule from which the body derives its energy. It is constructed from one Adenosine molecule and three phosphate molecules and referred to as ATP.

Aldosterone – is a hormone that causes the body to retain sodium.

Amino Acid – the 20 building blocks of proteins. There are 8 essential amino acids the body can not produce.

Amylase – is a digestive enzyme located in the salivary glands and pancreas. It is secreted in the mouth and small intestines to break down polysaccharides into oligosaccharides.

Anabolism – building up of tissue, either muscle tissue or fat stores.

Atrophy – a shrinking of muscle due to lack of use, disease, or injury.

Basal Metabolic Rate – the amount of calories a person needs in 24 hours doing absolutely nothing. This energy is the energy required to sustain muscle and maintain regular body functions / reactions.

Branched Chain Amino Acids (BCAA) – Leucine, isoleucine and valine. These amino acids are found in all animal source protein foods (chicken, meat and fish) and are also found in high concentrations in milk, cheese, yogurt and eggs.

Blood Sugar Levels – The amount of sugar (glucose) in your blood. 100 mg of glucose in 100 cubic centimeters of blood represents the normal range. Blood sugar levels dictate whether insulin or glucagons is released from the pancreas.

Brown Rice – A complex carbohydrate high in fiber and which increases blood sugar (glucose levels) slowly.

Caffeine – A drug that stimulates the nervous system. Caffeine stimulates lipase, an enzyme that allows fat to be mobilized and used as energy.

Calcium – is a mineral that promotes strong bones and teeth. Calcium also plays an integral part in the muscle contraction sequence.

Calorie – is a unit of measurement of the amount of heat it takes to raise the temperature of 1 liter of water 1 degree centigrade.

Carbohydrates – the body's preferred source of energy. Carbohydrates are converted to glucose (blood sugar) and also glycogen (stored blood sugar), stored in the liver and muscle. Carbohydrates are the main fuel source for resistance training.

Carbohydrate Metabolism – the breakdown of carbohydrates by amylase into glucose.

Carbon Dioxide –the by product of energy metabolism. It is exchanged for oxygen in the lungs at tiny sacs called alveoli. After exchange takes place, it is released, during exhalation.

Catabolic State – A state of muscle loss. The body begins to feed and maintain itself by the breakdown of protein stores located within the muscle.

Catabolism – A muscle wasting / destroying process that occurs due to stress producing (increased cortisol levels), insufficient calories, insufficient macronutrients.

Cellulose – An insoluble fiber. It is found in the outer coverings (skins) of fruits and vegetables.

Cholesterol – A type of lipid (fatty substance) that build up within body tissues.

Complete Protein – A protein that contains all nine essential amino acids.

Co-enzyme – Small molecules that assist enzymes to perform their functions.

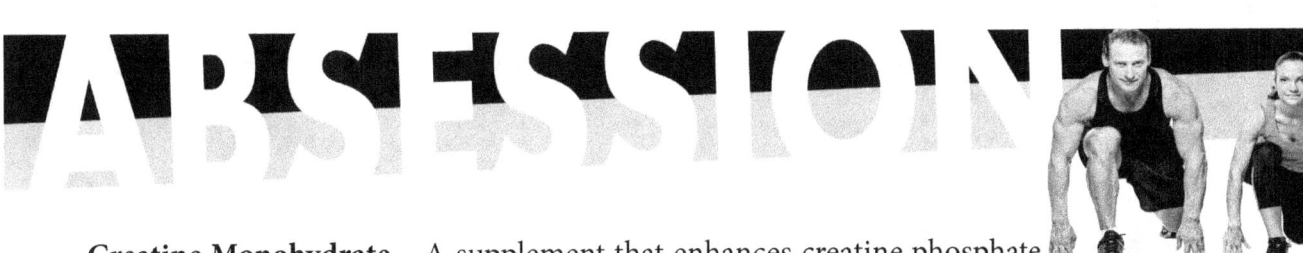

Creatine Monohydrate – A supplement that enhances creatine phosphate levels in the body. Increased levels allow more ATP to be made quicker.

Cortisol – A stress hormone that raises blood glucose levels by catabolizing body protein.

Creatine Phosphate – Energy compound that aids in the resynthesization of ATP.

Dietary Fatty Acid (DFA) – Essential fatty acids obtained by external sources because the body is unable to produce them. These fats are gamma linoleic acid and alpha linoleic acid.

Diet – **is** Latin for "Way of Life". In today's society, it is used to describe all the foods a person eats on a daily basis.

Dietary Fiber – Non-digestible food substances found primarily in plants. Fiber may lower blood glucose levels by slowing the absorption of carbohydrates into the blood.

Di-peptide – The term for 2 amino acids joined together.

Disaccharide – A simple sugar composed of two monosaccharide.

Ectomorph – is one of 3 somatotypes. Ectomorphs are lean, small bone structure and struggle to put on muscle or fat.

Electrolytes – Salts that allow electrical transfer of currents in the body. The 3 electrolytes are potassium, chloride and sodium. Potassium is pivotal in the muscle contraction process.

Endomorph – A somatotype. Endomorphs have large frames; carry some muscle mass but a significant fat mass.

Energy – Derived from the macronutrients carbohydrates, fats and protein. One gram of carbohydrates and protein yield 4 calories, while one gram of fat yields 9 calories.

Essential Amino Acids – Can not be made by the body and must be consumed in the diet for normal growth. There are 8 essential Amino Acids.

Essential Fatty Acids – These are the fatty acids that the body can not make and must get through the food consumed.

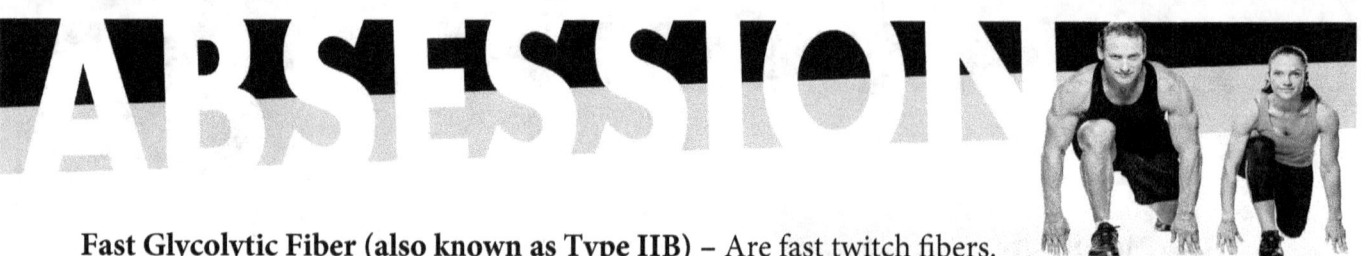

Fast Glycolytic Fiber (also known as Type IIB) – Are fast twitch fibers. They fatigue easily and generate great force. These fibers are stimulated during repetitions of 4-6 /8 done to failure or near failure, greatest potential for muscle hypertrophy.

Fast Oxidative Glycolytic Fiber (also known as Type IIA) – Are fast twitch fibers that carry properties of both Type IIB fibers and Type I fibers (Slow twitch fibers). These fibers are stimulated during repetitions of 8-12 repetitions done to failure or near failure.

Fat – An essential macronutrient that provides energy, insulation and protection to vital organs. Fat is stored in the body either as subcutaneous fat or visceral fat.

Fat soluble vitamins – Are vitamins that stored predominantly in the body's fat and liver. These vitamins include A, D, E and K.

Fatty acid – The building block of fats, also is the major energy producer for low intensity, long duration aerobic activities. Once oxidized and hydrolyzed, fatty acids enter into the cell's mitochondria to facilitate energy production.

Filaments – (also known as contractile filaments) Contractile proteins Actin and Myosin which comprise the myofibril. These proteins grow larger in size (hypertrophy) due to resistance training.

Free Radicals – Are oxygen atoms / molecules that are unstable in nature. These atoms are produced during exercise and have a damaging effect on the body with evidence pointing to their promotion of diabetes and other immune system maladies.

Fructose – A type of sugar found in fruit. When it is bonded together with glucose it forms the disaccharide sucrose, very high on the glycemic index rating table.

Galactose – Is a type of simple sugar, when combined with glucose it forms a disaccharide lactose.

Gluconeogenesis – "The new beginning of sugar." When the body is deprived of carbohydrates, the body will take non-carbohydrate sources like protein, amino acids and lean body tissue converting them into glucose.

Glucose – The sugar that is found in the blood. It is used exclusively by cells for fuel. Carbohydrate foods are broken down into glucose to be used as fuel.

Glycemic Index – A rating system to monitor how quickly blood glucose levels rise after consumption of a particular food. The Glycemic Index was initially devised to monitor blood glucose in diabetics.

Glycogen – The body's stored form of carbohydrates. The body will store glycogen as either liver glycogen or as muscle glycogen so it can be used as fuel when needed.

Glycolysis – the breakdown of sugar leading to the formation of pyruvate, the initial step in the anaerobic Glycolysis energy system.

High Density Lipoprotein – is a form of cholesterol that removes some fats from the blood. Exercise increases HDL, which has desirable effects on the body.

Hyperplasia – Increase in the number of cells in a tissue.

Hypertrophy – Increase in the size of a tissue due to an increase in cell size. **Hypogly-cemia** – A deficiency of sugar in the blood, is a direct result of too much insulin released by the pancreas or by prolonged exercise sessions.

Insulin – A storage hormone secreted by the pancreas whenever blood glucose levels exceed the body's normal range. Insulin drives glucose out of the blood and into the muscle cells to form muscle glycogen.

Iron – Is a mineral needed in small amounts to aid in the body's functions and helps the formation of red blood cells.

Isoleucine – Is one of the three branched chain amino acids. Amino acids can be used as fuel by muscles during training sessions. BCAA's help avoid muscle catabolism.

Krebs Cycle – A repeating process involving high energy intermediates that generate ATP.

Lactic Acid – A by product of anaerobic energy production, accumulating during short term high intensity exercise.

Lactic Acid System – An energy production system that uses carbohydrates and ultimately glucose or stored glycogen without the need of oxygen.

Low Density Lipoprotein – Plasma complex of lipids and proteins that contain more cholesterol and triglycerides and less protein. High LDL is associated with contributing to coronary heart disease.

Leucine –Branched Chain Amino Acid. It increases the rate of muscle synthesis by increasing of insulin levels in the pancreas, also used as a fuel to generate Adenosine Tri-Phosphate.

Lipase – is an enzyme that breaks down dietary fat into fragments.

Lipid – Fat or fat-like substances

Lipoprotein – transporter of fat through the body, Composed of protein, fat and cholesterol.

Medium Chain Triglycerides (MCT) – Shorter length fats, used as an immediate energy source and produces ketone bodies which can be used as a fuel source.

Mesomorph – Body type that is comprised of mainly muscle, bone and connective tissues with very little bodyfat, predisposed to lean muscle mass gains with little bodyfat accumulation.

Metabolism – Processes by which the body produces energy derived from the consumption of fuel (food).

Monosaccharide – Simple sugars (ex. Blood sugar and a constituent of fruit.)

Minerals – Inorganic substances needed in small amounts to aid in the body's biochemical reactions.

Myosin –The thicker of the 2 contractile proteins, which resides within the myofibril of the muscle.

Non- essential Amino Acid – An amino acid that can be synthesized by the body and does not need to be obtained externally.

Nutrient – Mandatory substances required for health and body growth, classified into Macro (needed in large amounts) and Micro (needed in small amounts). Macronutrients include carbohydrates, protein, fats and water. Micronutrients include minerals and vitamins.

Nutrition – Is the study of foods and their affect on the body.

Omega 3 Fatty Acid – Healthy fat found in cold water fish, possessive positive health effects by increasing muscle cell receptor sites' sensitivity, making it easier for insulin to drive nutrients into muscle cells.

Pepsin – Enzyme that breaks protein into peptides.

Phosphorous – Mineral needed for production of ATP. It also metabolizes carbohydrates, fats and proteins.

Polypeptide – Long chain of amino acids.

Potassium – A mineral found inside muscle. It is required for muscle contraction.

Proteins – Food substances constructed of amino acids. Functions include repair and growth of tissue, hormone production and certain enzyme functions.

Pyruvate – The result of the breakdown of one molecule of sugar ($C_6H_{12}O_6$). Pyruvate is C_3 and is ultimately used to produce ATP.

Ratio of Energy – Amount of fat calories in relationship to a person's total caloric intake.

Relative Body Fat – Amount of fat relative to a person's muscle tissue.

Saturated Fatty Acids – Fatty acids that have the maximum number of hydrogen atoms, found primarily in animal sources, solid at room temperature.

Slow Twitch Fiber – Muscle fiber characterized by its slow contraction speed, high capacity for aerobic Glycolysis also known as Red, Type II Fibers.

Starch (also known as polysaccharides) – Form of complex carbohydrate. Consumption of complex Carbs produces a slower spike in insulin levels as opposed to simple Carbs.

Subcutaneous Fat – Fat found under the skin, as opposed to visceral fat which is packed densely around the body's organs.

Sugar (Carbohydrates) – Which are classified as either simple or complex.

Thiamine – Known as Vitamin B-1, aids in the release of energy from carbohydrates.

Triglyceride – Storage form of fat consisting of one glycerol molecule and three fatty acids. Triglycerides are the major fuel source for low intensity, long duration aerobic activities.

Tri-peptide – Chain of 3 amino acids

Unsaturated Fatty Acids – Fats found in nuts and vegetable oils, liquid at room temperature. Classified as polyunsaturated and monounsaturated fats.

Valine – One of the BCAA's that can be used as fuel when working anaerobically.

Vitains - Organic compound needed in small amounts by the body. Controls metabolic processes and can not be synthesized by the body.

Vitamin A – Fat soluble vitamin found in animal tissues. Aids in growth, healthy skin and facilitates other bodily metabolic functions.

Vitamin B – Water soluble vitamins that includes B1, B2, B3, B5, B6 B12, Biotin and folic acid. Found in whole grains, aids in metabolism of nutrients consumed.

Vitamin C – Water soluble vitamin, is also known as Ascorbic Acid. Found in Citrus Fruits. Forms collagen, aids in muscle recovery, fights free radicals and supports thyroid functions.

Vitamin D – Fat soluble vitamin found predominantly in milk and milk products. Aids in the production of strong bones, supports nervous system and heart functions.

Vitamin E – Fat soluble vitamin found in eggs and meat sources, strong anti-oxidant that improves the body's glucose efficiency.

Vitamin F – Water soluble vitamin also known as folic acid, produces Red and White Blood Cells.

Vitamin K – Fat soluble vitamin found in vegetables and milk products which assist in the clotting of blood.

Water Soluble Vitamins – vitamins that dissolve in water that include: Vitamins C, B1, B2, Niacin, B6, Folacin and B12.

Appendix / Forms

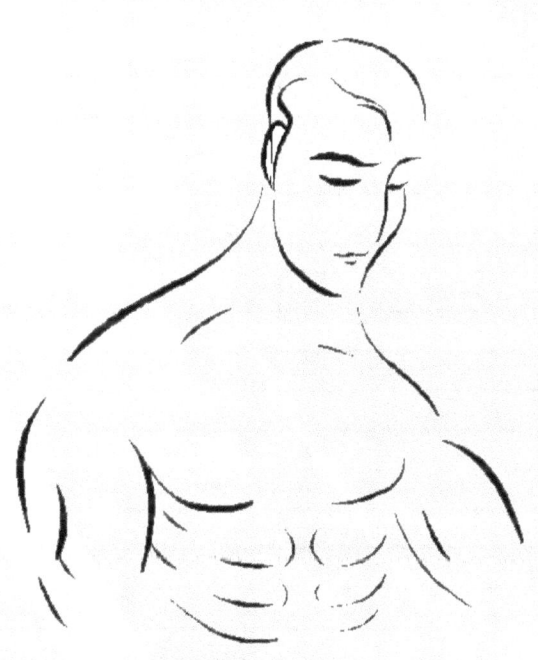

ABSESSION

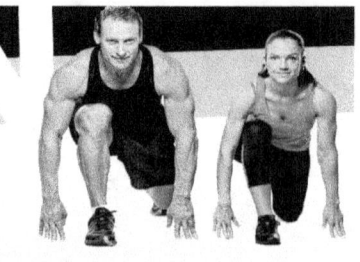

NUTRITION JOURNAL

Week: _____ Day: _____ Date: _____

MEAL	FOOD CHOICES	CALORIES	CARBO-HYDRATES	PROTEIN	FAT
1					
2					
3					
4					
5					
6					

NOTES:

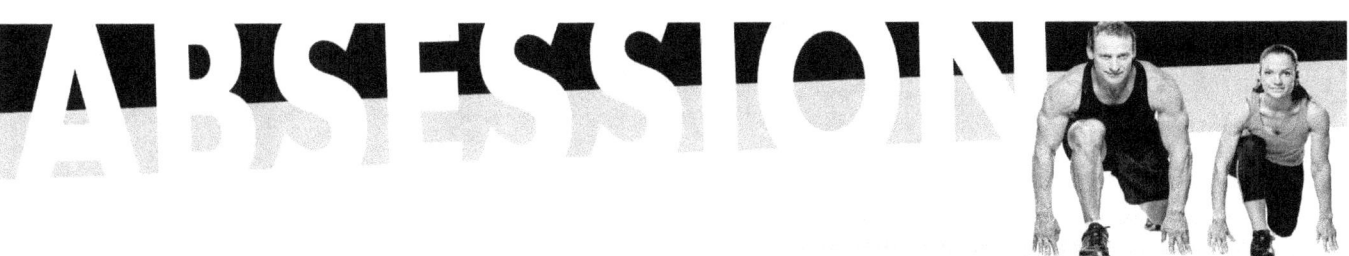

AB SESSION

Name: _____ Date: _____ Day of Week: _____ Motivtion_____

Hi / Med / Low

RESISTANCE TRAINING LOG					
		Set 1	Set 2	Set 3	Set 4
BODYPART	**EXERCISE**	WEIGHT ------------ Reps	WEIGHT ------------ Reps	WEIGHT ------------ Reps	WEIGHT ------------ Reps
CHEST					
BACK					
SHOULDERS					
LEGS (QUADS)					
LEGS (HAMSTRINGS)					
BICEPS					
TRICEPS					
CALVES					
TRAPS					
ABDOMINALS					
LOW BACK					
NOTES:					

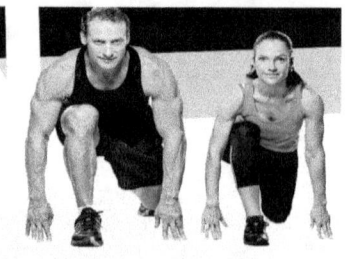

ABSESSION

Cardiovascular Exercise Log

Day	Mode	Intensity[1]	Heart Rate[2]	Start Time	Finish Time

1) Intensity includes speed, % incline etc.   2) Heart rate at the end of exercise

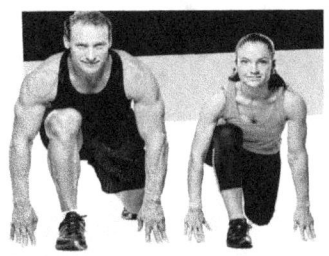

ASSESSMENT LOG

Week	Weight	Body Fat %	Resting Heart Rate	Waist Measurement (Men)	Hip Measurement (Women)
Week 1					
Week 2					
Week 3					
Week 4					
Week 5					
Week 6					
Week 7					
Week 8					
Week 9					
Week 10					
Week 11					
Week 12					

NOTES:

EXERCISE SUMMARIES

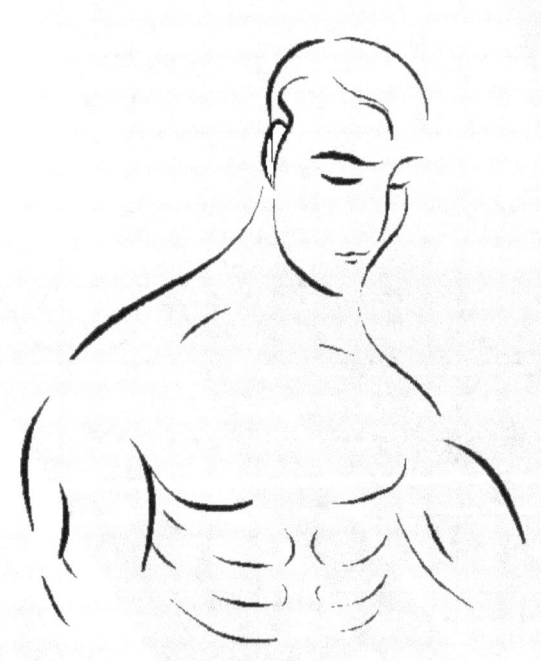

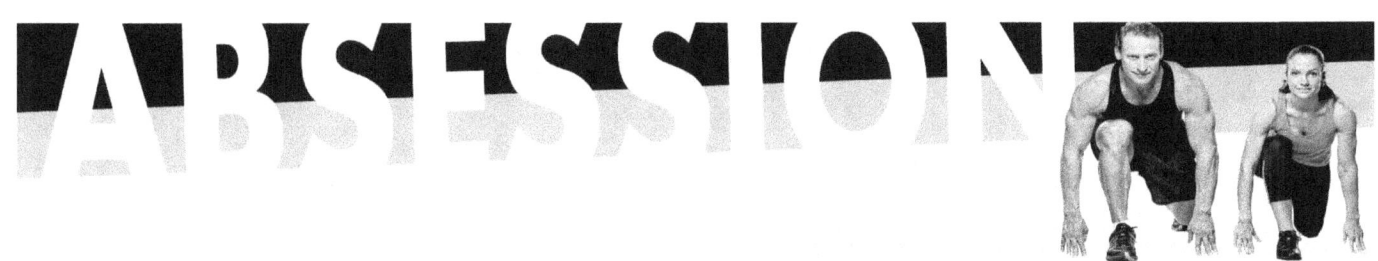

The following exercise descriptions are mentioned in Chapter 5. There are many other exercises, but the following are major multi joint exercises that work major muscles of the body.

Caution: Please consult your physician before starting this or any workout program.

Reminder: The following exercises will describe the concentric (or the positive) portion of the exercise and the eccentric (or the negative) portion of the exercise. The concentric portion should be performed at a speed of two seconds, while exhaling and the eccentric portion of the exercise should be performed at a speed of four seconds while inhaling.

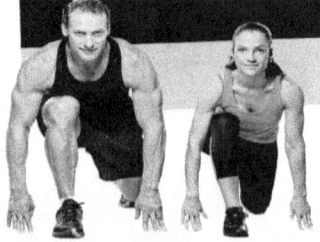

FLAT BENCH PRESS
BARBELL / DUMBBELL

Primary muscle(s): Pectoralis Major
Synergistic muscle(s): Triceps brachii, Anterior Deltoid

DESCRIPTION:

- Lie on flat bench with feet planted firmly on floor

- Grasp bar slightly wider than shoulder width apart with thumbs wrapped around bar

- Lift bar (or have spotter assist you) off of uprights and balance bar over chin area with arms fully extended

- Lower bar while inhaling to a four second count

- Bar should travel in a path of an arc until it makes (light) contact with chest area

- Elbows should be flared outward (to maximize pectoralis stimulation) at approximately 45°

- Drive bar back to start position (without bouncing bar off of chest)

- Exhale during (concentric) positive portion

- Positive (concentric) portion should take 2 seconds

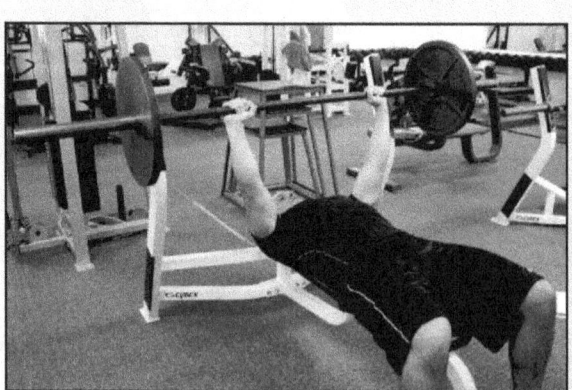 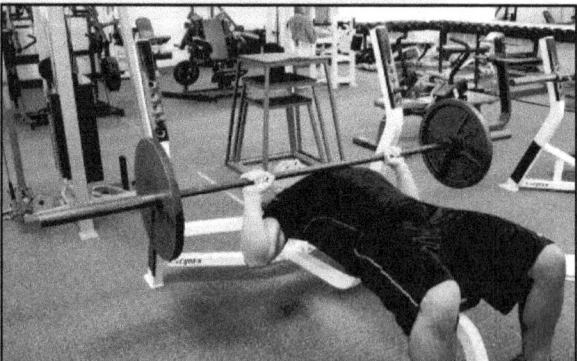

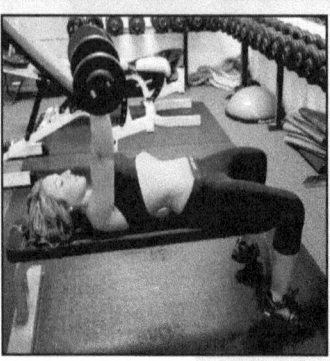 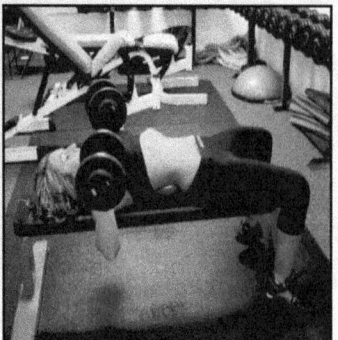

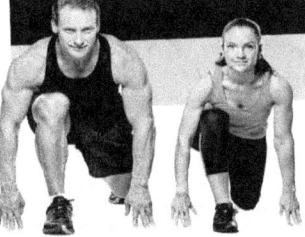

BARBELL / DUMBBELL

Primary muscle(s): Pectoralis Major
Synergistic muscle(s): Triceps brachii, Anterior Deltoid

DESCRIPTION:

- Set bench at approximately 30° (any more of an incline places more focus on shoulders)

- Follow same timing for concentric / eccentric portions of lift as flat bench press

- Emphasizes upper 1/3 of pectoralis major (chest)

- Path of bar travels straight up and down as opposed to in an arc (as in the flat bench press)

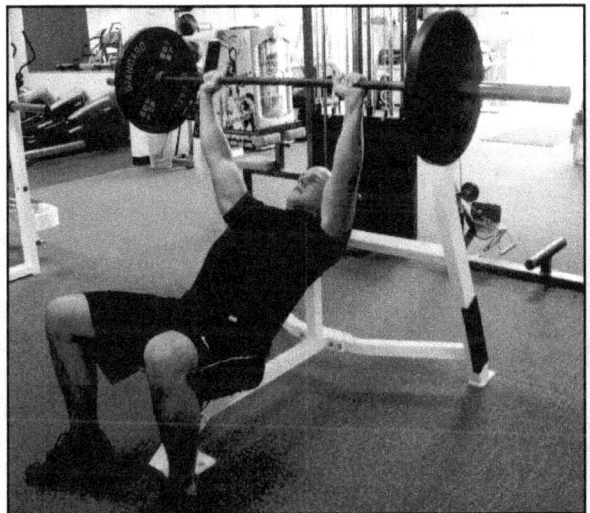
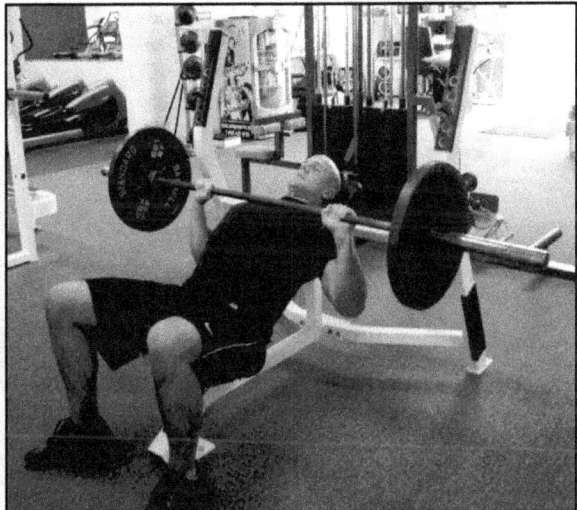

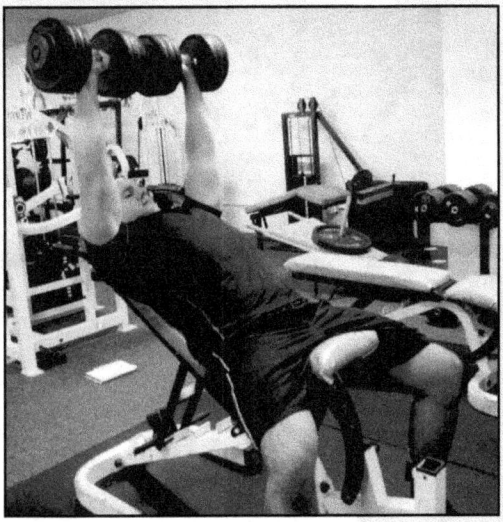
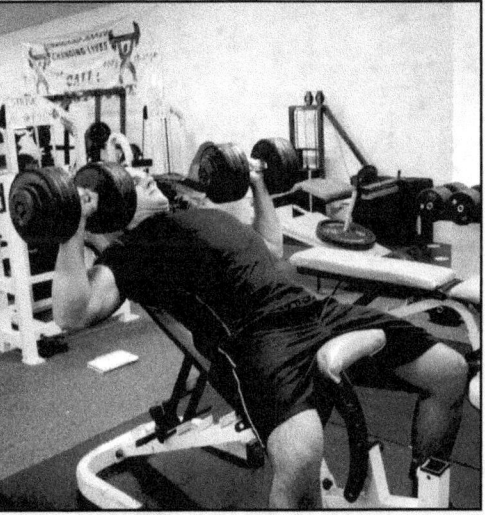

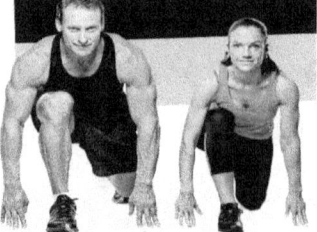

BARBELL / DUMBBELL

Primary muscle(s): Pectoralis Major
Synergistic muscle(s): Triceps brachii, Anterior Deltoid

DESCRIPTION:

- Emphasizes mid to lower pectoralis major (chest)

- Line of motion will be from just below chest area straight up and down

- Bench should be kept at no more than 30° angle

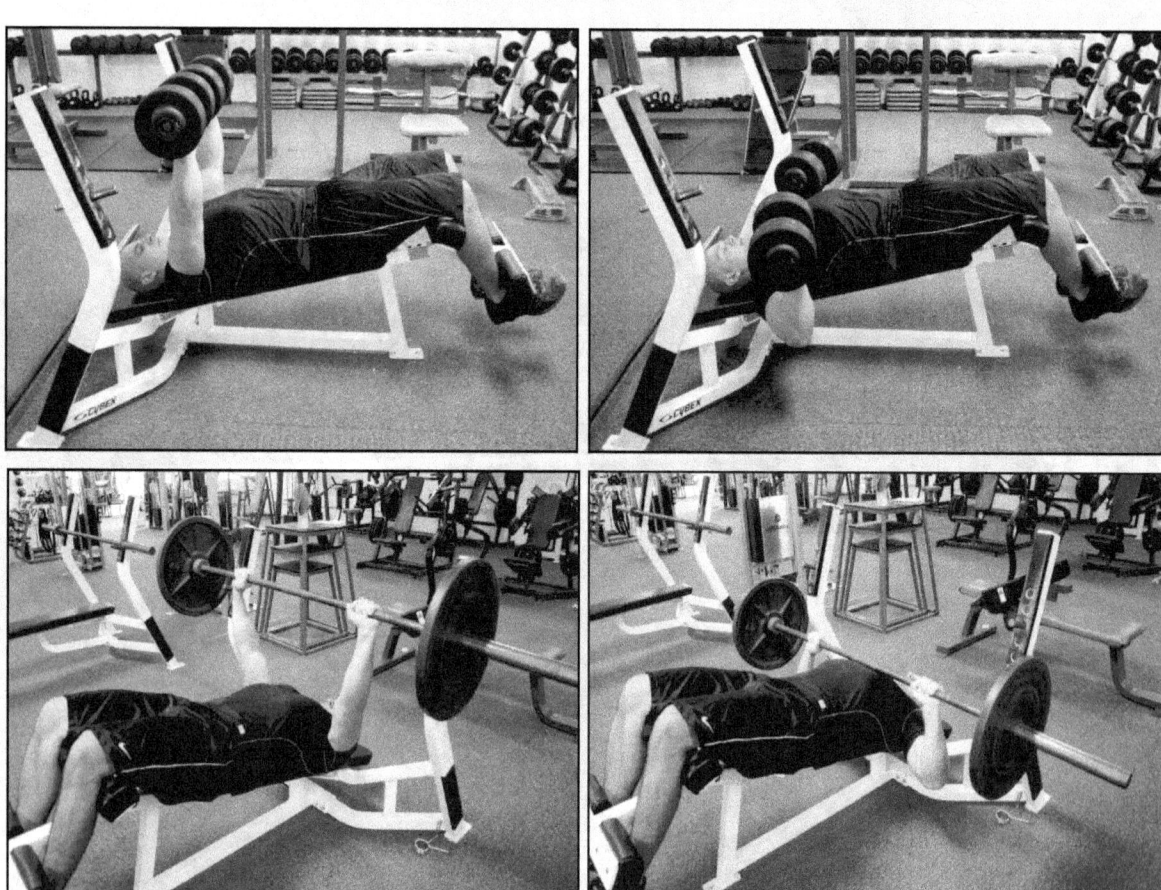

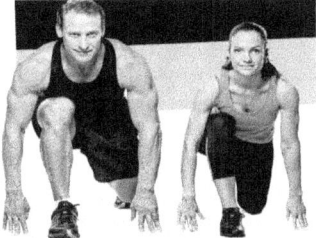

PARALLEL BARS

Primary muscle(s): Pectoralis Major

Synergistic muscle(s): Triceps brachii, Anterior Deltoid

DESCRIPTION:

- Begin by supporting bodyweight with arms straight between parallel bars
- For chest- keep body lean forward with elbows flared out
- Bend elbows and lower body
- Lower body until elbows form a 90° angle
- Push torso back to start position by extending arms
- Do not extend arms to full lock out
- Repeat for desired number of repetitions

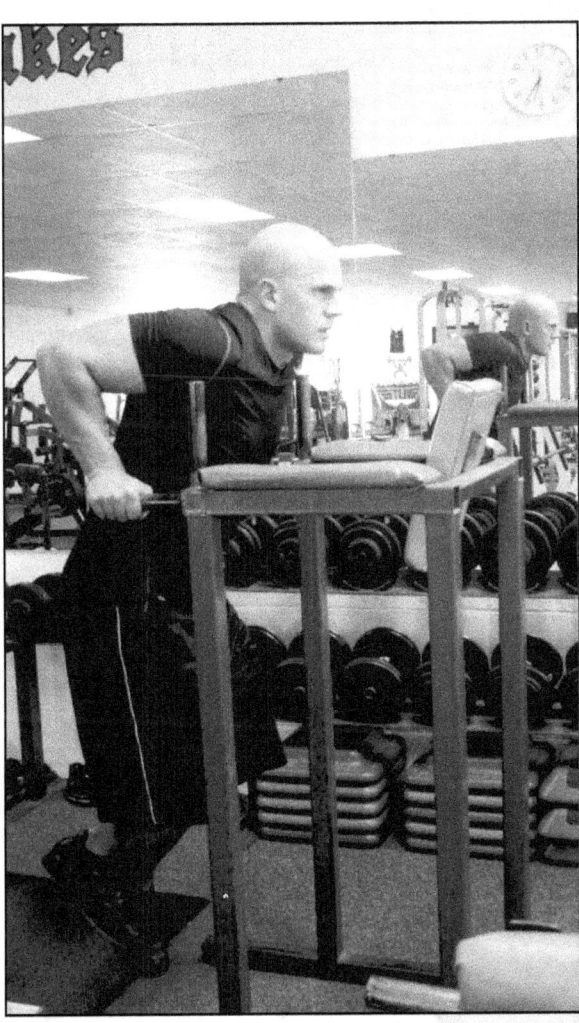
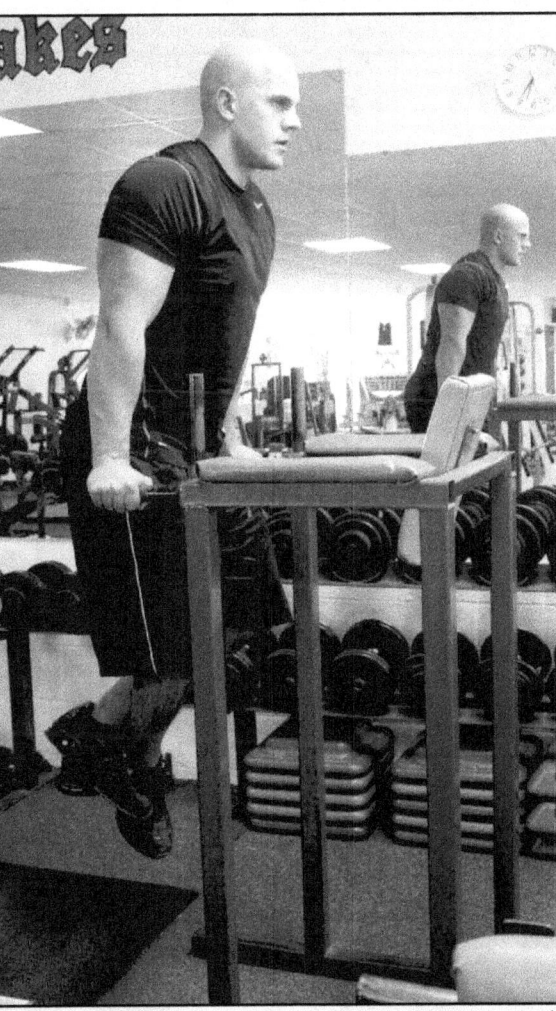

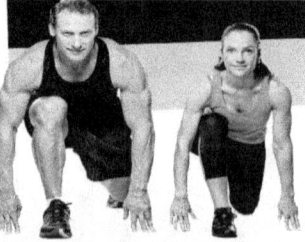

PULLLUPS
PULL UP BAR

Primary muscle(s): Latissimus Dorsi
Synergistic muscle(s): Biceps Brachii, Brachialis,
Brachioradialis, Teres Minor,
Posterior Deltoid

DESCRIPTION

- Grasp chin up bar with an overhand grip slightly wider than shoulder width apart
- Retract scapula
- Pull body up in a vertical line, until chin reaches bar
- Slowly return to start position without releasing tension on muscle
- Repeat for desired number of repetitions

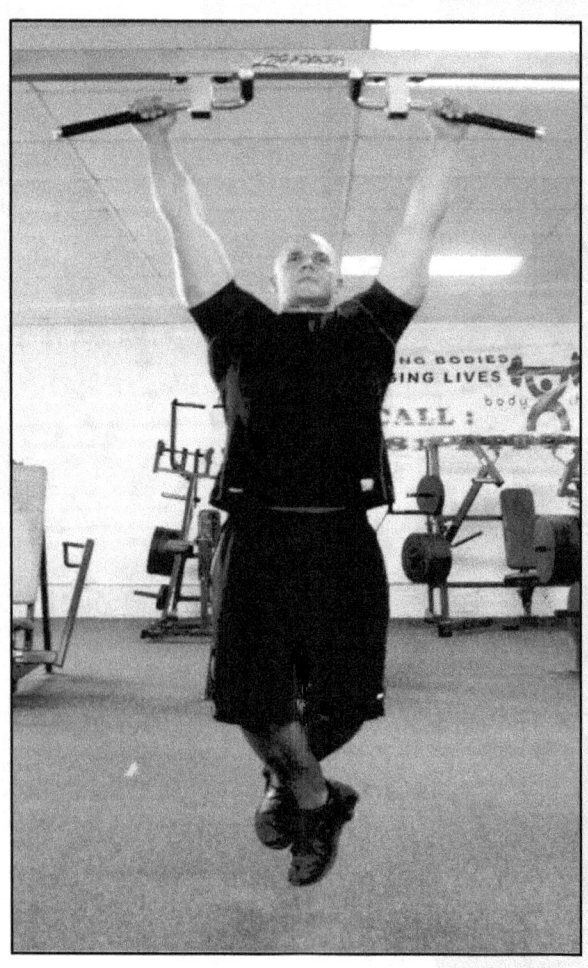
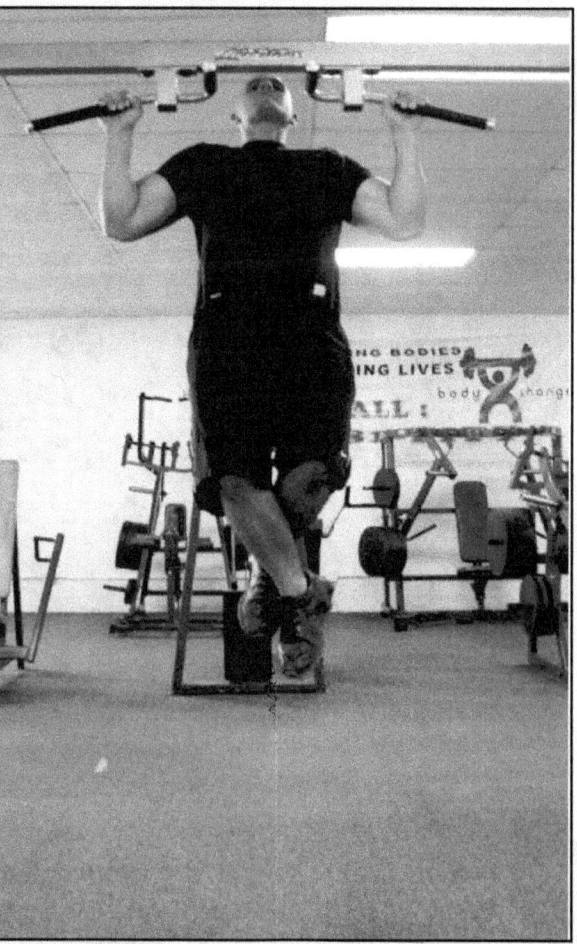

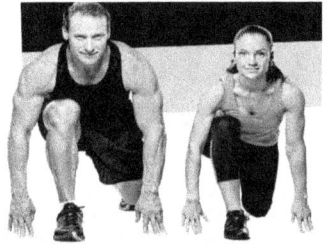

OVERHEAD CABLE LAT PULL DOWN

Primary muscle(s): Latissimus Dorsi
Synergistic muscle(s): Biceps Brachii, Brachialis,
Brachioradialis, Teres Minor,
Posterior Deltoid

DESCRIPTION:

- Position yourself underneath an overhead cable pull down station and secure yourself underneath the knee pads.
- Keep feet flat on the floor
- Grab bar slightly wider than shoulder width apart with an overhand grip
- Retract scapula
- For the concentric portion of the lift, pull the bar down until it makes light contact with the upper chest area
- The concentric phase (positive) should take 2 seconds and you should exhale
- The eccentric phase (negative) should take 4 seconds and you should inhale
- During the eccentric phase the exerciser should allow the bar to return to the starting point
- Do not allow scapula to protract (this will take tension off the working muscle)

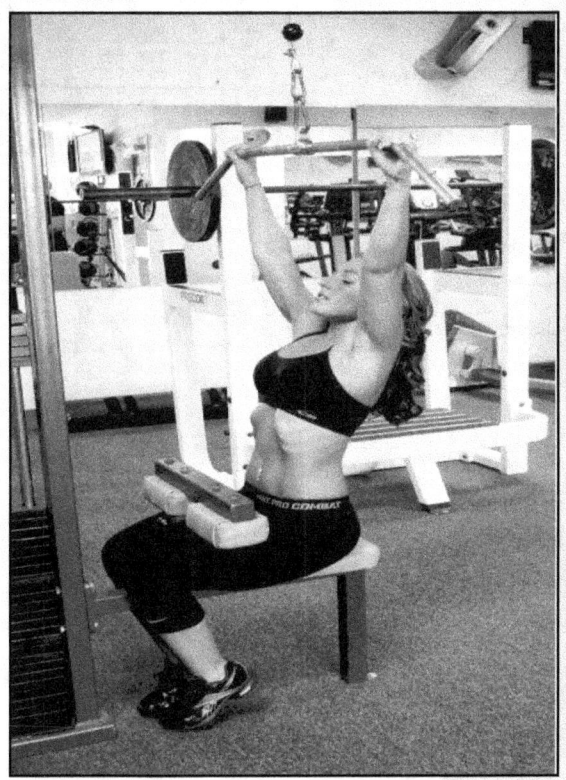
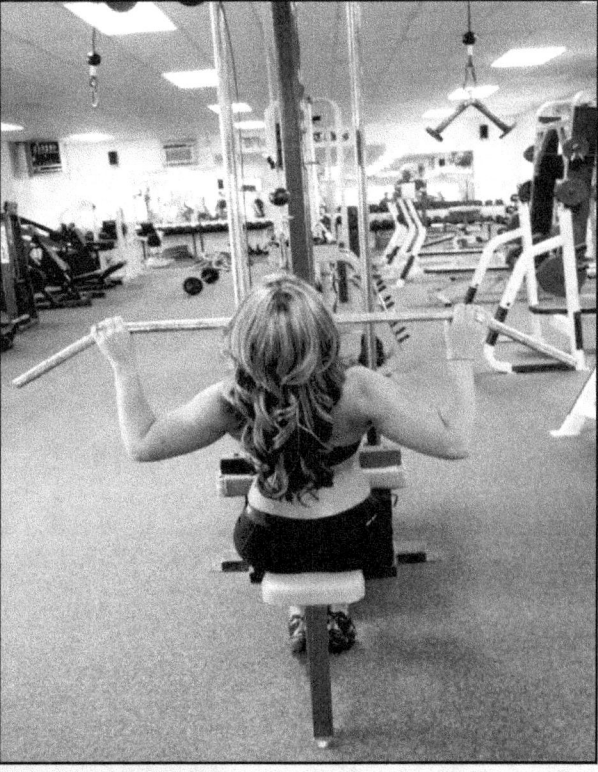

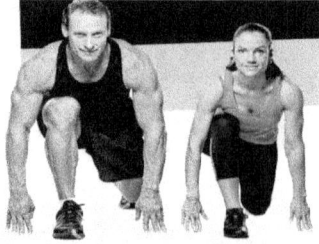

BARBELL

Primary muscle(s): Latissimus Dorsi Synergistic
muscle(s): Biceps Brachii, Brachialis,

Brachioradialis, Teres Minor,

Posterior Deltoid

DESCRIPTION:

- Grasp bar using an overhand grip slightly wider than shoulder width apart (you may also opt for an underhand grip)
- Keep feet shoulder width apart
- Bend at hips, maintaining a neutral arch in back while keeping knees bent
- Retract scapula
- Initiating movement through the arms, pull bar upward until it touches abdomen
- Keep upper body not moving
- Lower weight on the eccentric to start position

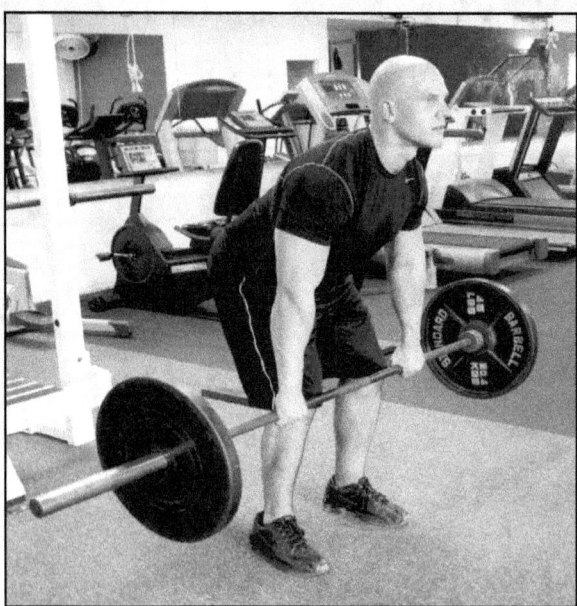
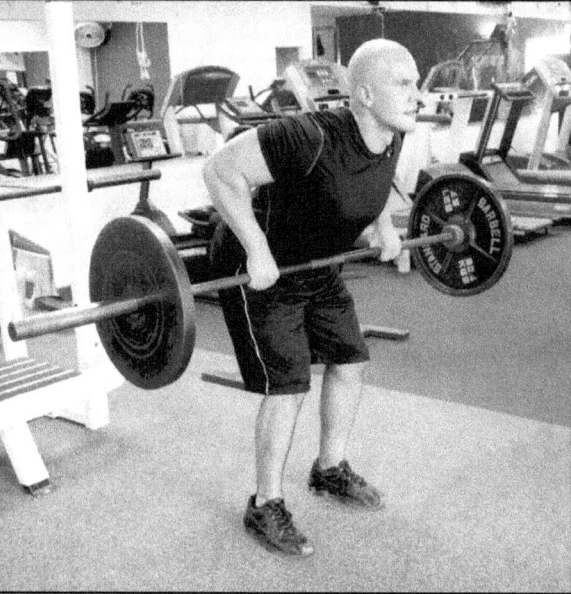

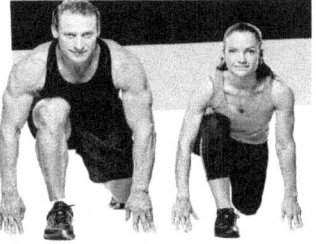

BARBELL

Primary muscle(s): Erector Spinae, Gluteus Maximus, Vastus Lateralis, Vastus Intermedius, Vastus Medialis, Rectus Femoris, Biceps Femoris, Semitendinosus, Semimembranosus

DESCRIPTION:

- While bar is resting on floor, stand close to bar with feet directly underneath bar.
- Feet should be slightly wider than shoulder width apart.
- Squat down by bending through the hips until you are able to grasp bar in an alternated grip.
- The bar should be up against your shins.
- Keep head straight ahead and maintain a neutral arch in back.
- Begin by lifting through hips while driving through the heels of your feet.
- Once the bar clears the patella, drive hips forward.
- Continue driving hips until lifter reaches a fully erect position.
- Lifter should not over-exaggerate a backward lean at the top of movement (this will place stress on the lower back).
- You should exhale during the concentric and it should take two seconds.
- For eccentric portion of the lift, slowly return to starting position by lowering hips and

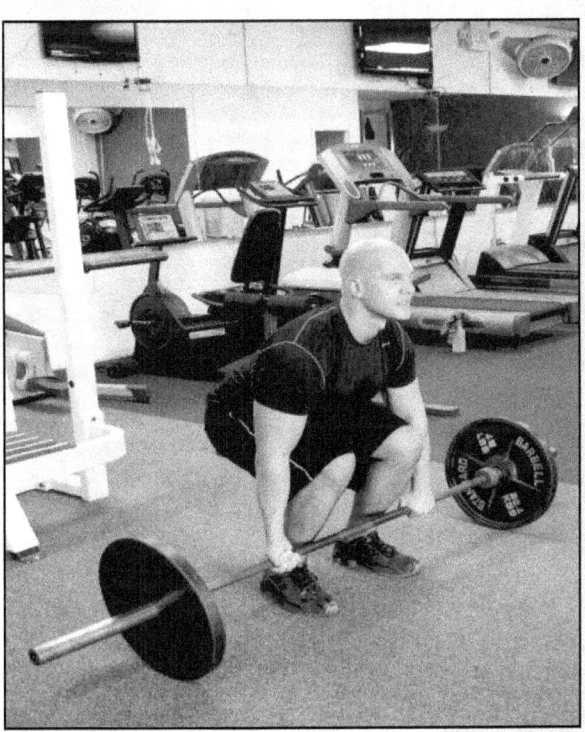
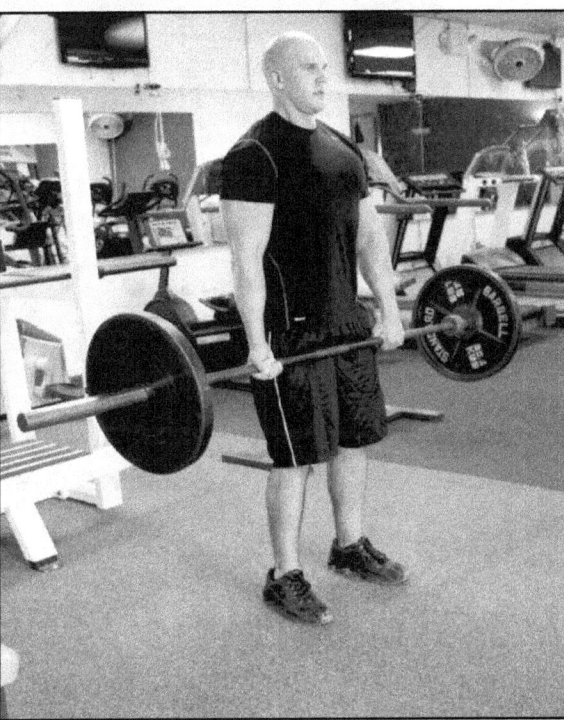

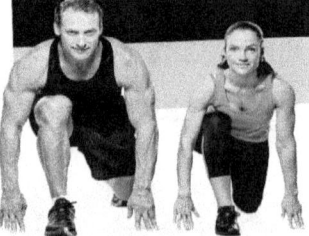

TBAR

Primary muscle(s): Rhomboids, Trapezius II,
Latissimus Dorsi,
Synergistic muscle(s): Biceps Brachii, Brachialis,
Brachioradialis, Teres Minor,
Posterior Deltoid

DESCRIPTION:

- Bend forward at hips, knees bent with back flat while maintaining a neutral arch in back.
- Grasp T bar handles in overhand grip.
- Raiser torso so that it is parallel to floor.
- Retract scapula.
- Arms should be extended but not locked out.

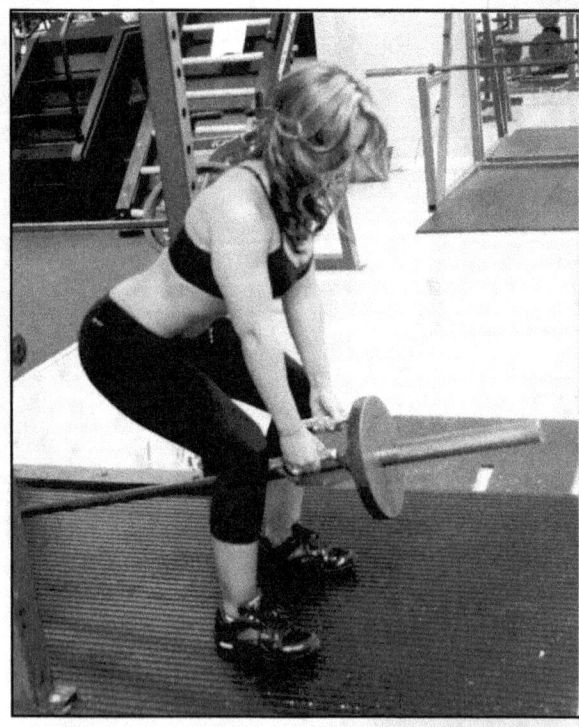
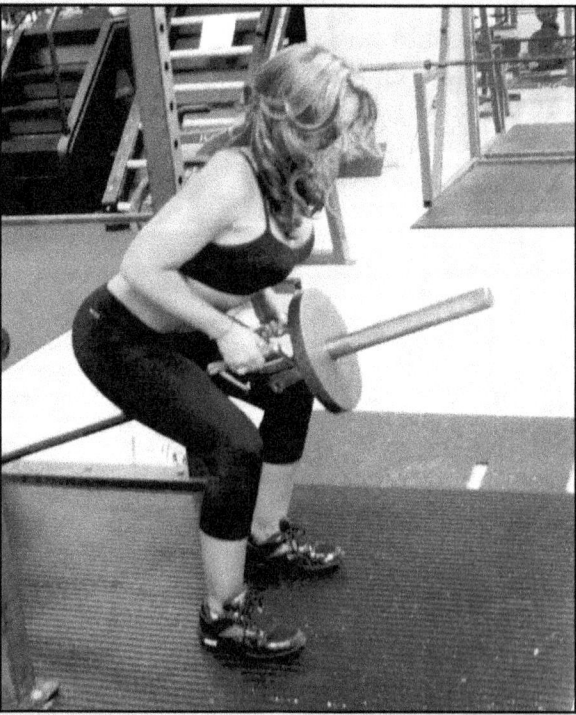

SEATED LOW CABLE PULLEY

Primary muscle(s): Rhomboids, Latissimus Dorsi, Trapezius II
Synergistic muscle(s): Biceps Brachii, Brachialis,
Brachioradialis, Teres Minor,
Posterior Deltoid

DESCRIPTION:

- Grasp seated pulley handle
- Place feet on foot rests
- Keep shoulders retracted
- Keep core tight
- Maintain slight bend in knees throughout exercise
- Pull handle in to abdominals while using Latissimus Dorsi to contract
- Keep elbows in close to body
- Return to start position, repeat for desired number of repetitions

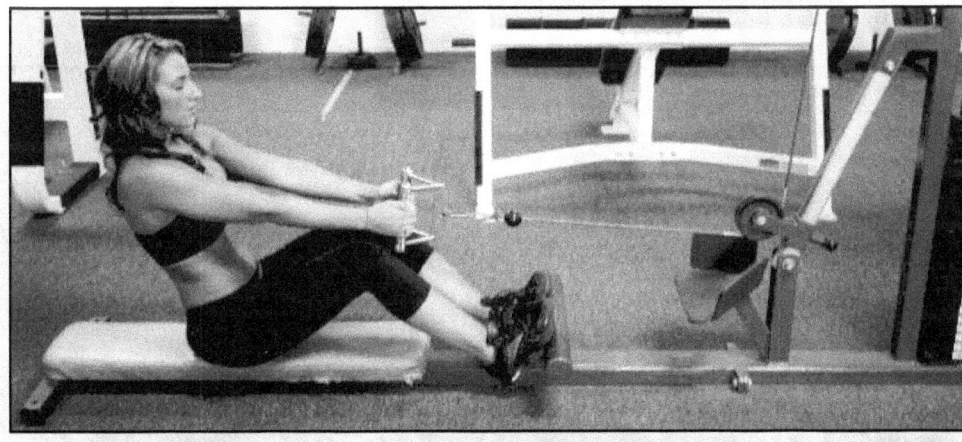

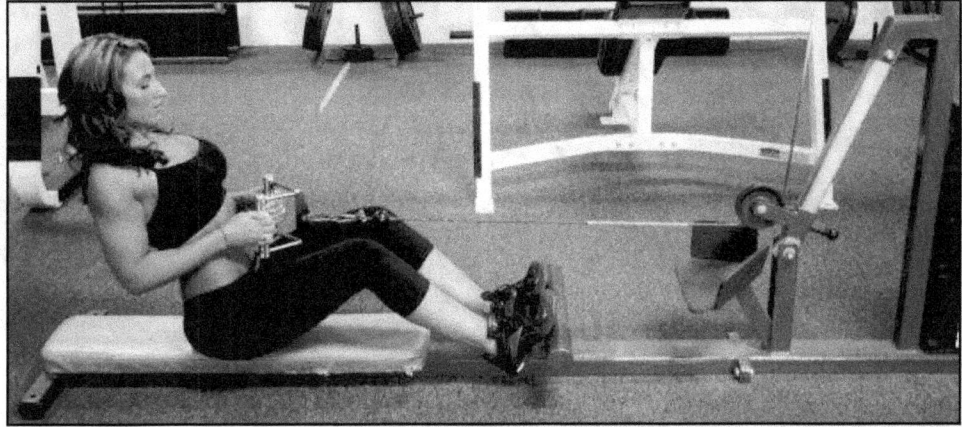

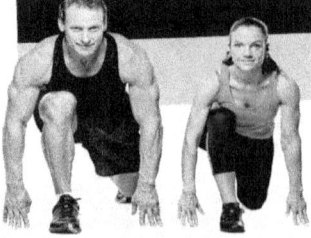

DUMBBELL, FLAT BENCH

Primary muscle(s): Latissimus Dorsi Synergistic
muscle(s): Biceps Brachii, Brachialis,
Brachioradialis, Teres Minor,
Posterior Deltoid

DESCRIPTION:

- Grasp dumbbell with right hand using an overhand grip (keep hand neutral)
- Rest opposite knee (left knee) on a flat bench
- Right leg should be straight with foot flat on floor
- Bend forward at hips, place left hand on bench for stability
- Upper torso should be parallel to floor
- Dumbbell should start at arm's length
- While keeping elbow close to upper torso, pull dumbbell upward until it reaches hip level
- Slowly lower dumbbell to start position
- Repeat for desired number of repetitions

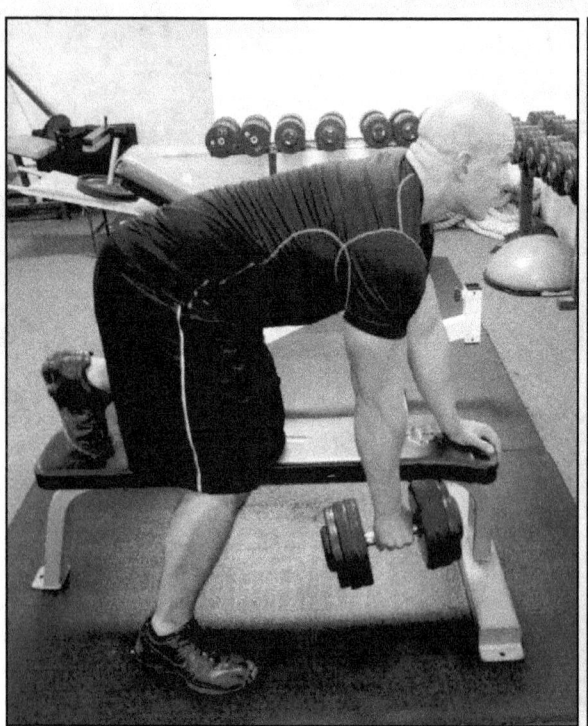
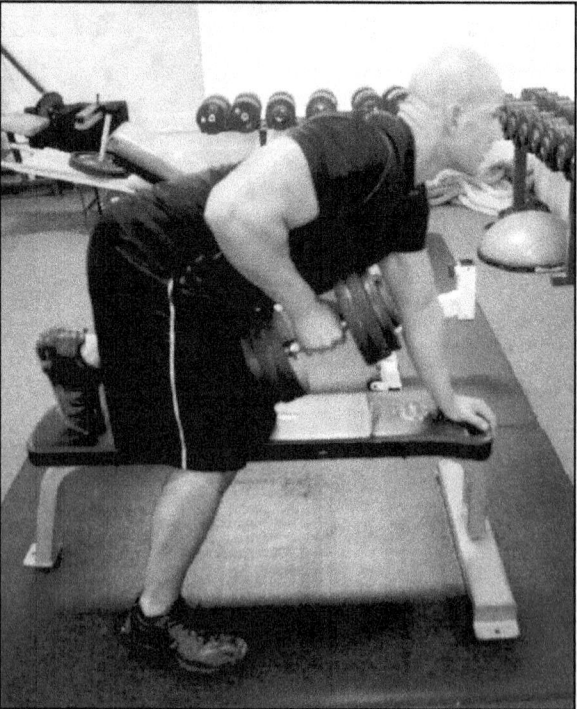

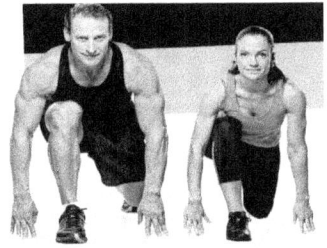

SEATED / STANDING BARBELL PRESS
BARBELL / DUMBBELLS

Primary muscle(s): Anterior, Medial & Poster Deltoids
Synergistic muscle(s): Triceps Brachii

DESCRIPTION:

- Stand or sit on a bench with back in contact with back support of chair
- Grasp bar using an overhand grip, slightly wider than shoulder width apart
- Remove bar from uprights with assistance from spotter
- Slowly slower the bar for the eccentric portion until elbows reside at a 90° angle
- Slowly press weight back until arms are at an extended, but not locked position
- Repeat for desired number of repetitions

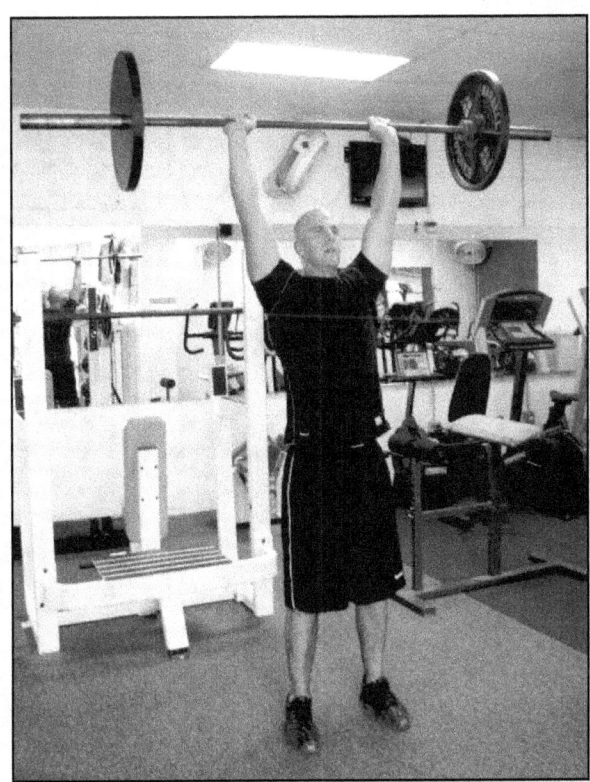
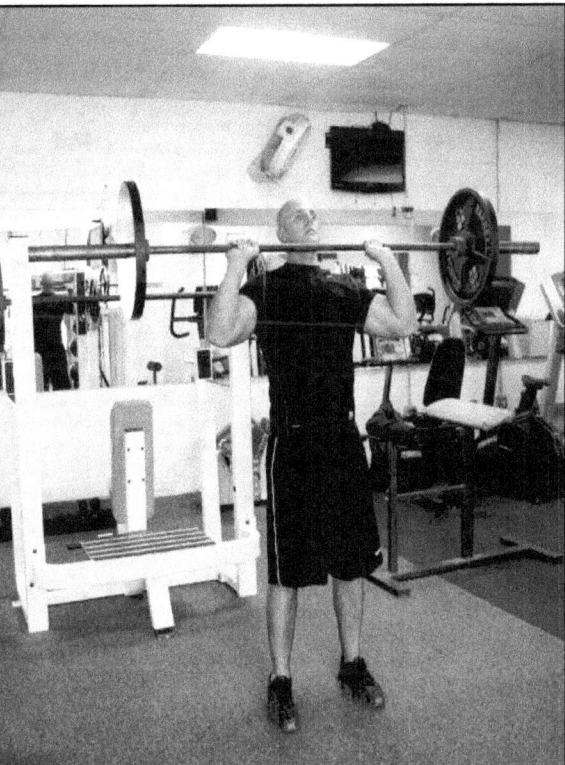

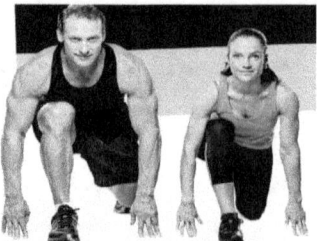

ABSESSION

BARBELL

Primary muscle(s): Medial Deltoid
Synergistic muscle(s): Trapezius I, Brachioradialis

DESCRIPTION:

- Keep back in a neutral, weightlifter's arch
- Keep knees bent, shoulders retracted
- Grasp barbell with overhand grip

(Hands slightly closer than hip width for focus on Trapezius, hands slightly wider than shoulder width apart for focus on medial deltoid)

- Hold barbell at arm's length with slight bend in elbows, bar should be at thigh level
- Begin the concentric portion of the exercise by raising bar (while staying close to your body) until it reaches chin level
- You want to initiate motion by raising elbows
- Low bar back to starting position for eccentric portion

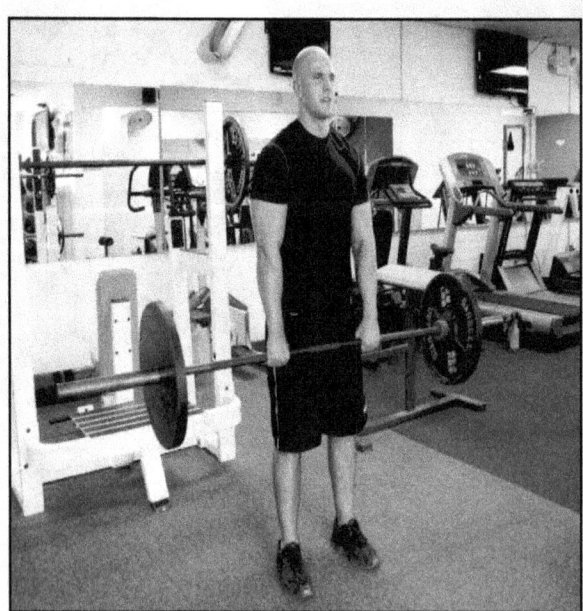
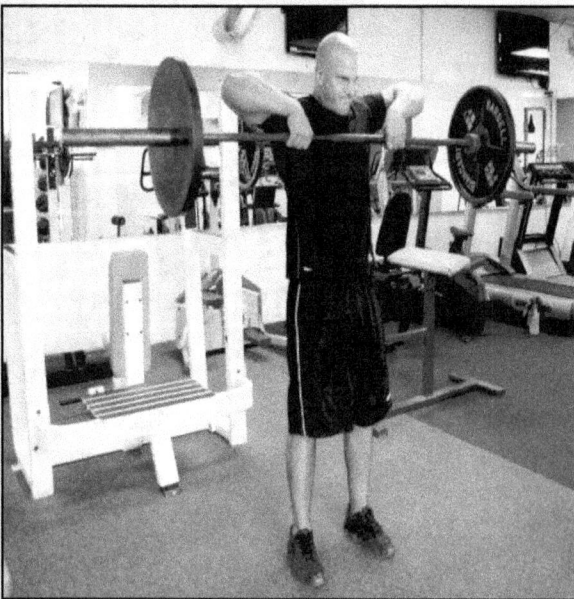

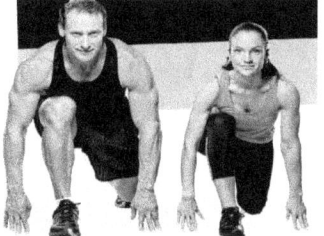

SQUAT

BARBELL / DUMBBELLS / SMITH MACHINE

Primary muscle(s): Quadriceps Group
Synergistic muscle(s): Gluteus Maximus,

Hamstring Group

DESCRIPTION:

- Grasp bar in an overhand grip slightly wider than shoulder width apart
- Feet should be slightly wider than hip width apart
- Retract scapula
- Place bar on the upper Trapezius (forming a platform for the bar)
- Roll elbows forward to lock bar onto the Trapezius area
- Stand up underneath bar and remove bar from squat rack uprights (with assistance from spotter)
- Slowly step back and away from the uprights
- Begin by sitting back with hips (this is to clear the area so the chest can move downward)
- Keep head forward and back neutral throughout lift
- Do not break knee toe line (allowing the knee to travel out in front of toes)
- Continue the eccentric portion of the lift until your hips are parallel to the floor
- You should form a 90° angle
- Begin the Concentric portion of the lift by driving upward through your heels and returning to the starting position
- Do not bounce at the bottom of the eccentric portion of the lift (this places unneeded stress on the patella)
- Do not lock out knees as the top of the movement (this will remove the tension from the working muscles and place unneeded stress on the patella)
- Repeat for desired number of repetitions

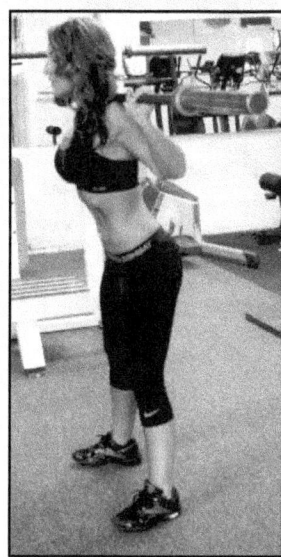
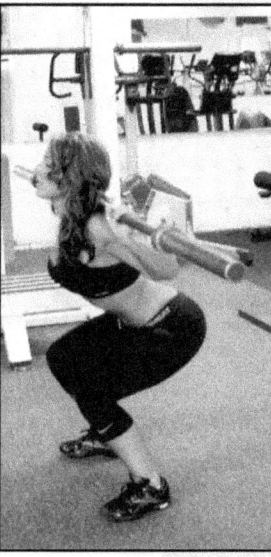
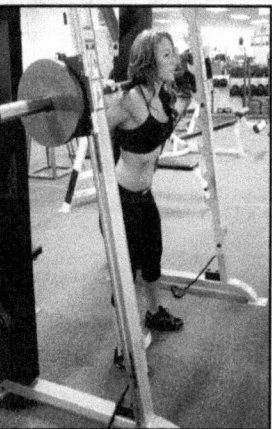
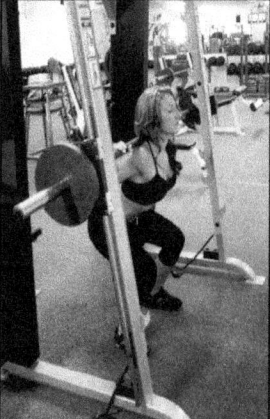

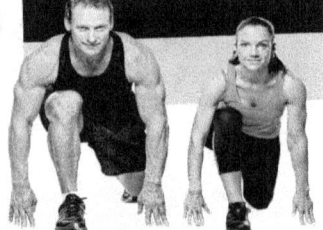

LEG PRESS MACHINE

Primary muscle(s): Quadriceps Group

Synergistic muscle(s): Gluteus Maximus, Hamstring Group

DESCRIPTION:

- Lie back on leg press machine
- Keep feet shoulder width apart on platform
- Knees should track directly over toes
- Maintain knee toe line and knee hip line that was discussed in the squat
- Slowly lift weight and rotate safety catches out of the way
- For the eccentric portion of the lift, slowly descend while inhaling
- Eccentric portion should take four seconds
- Do not bounce at bottom of the movement
- For the concentric portion of the lift, drive the weight back to starting position
- Drive through the heels
- Do not lock knees at top of motion (this will remove tension from the working muscle and place unneeded stress on the patella)
- The concentric portion of the lift should take two seconds
- Exhale during the concentric portion
- Once completing desired number of repetitions, return safeties to their locked position

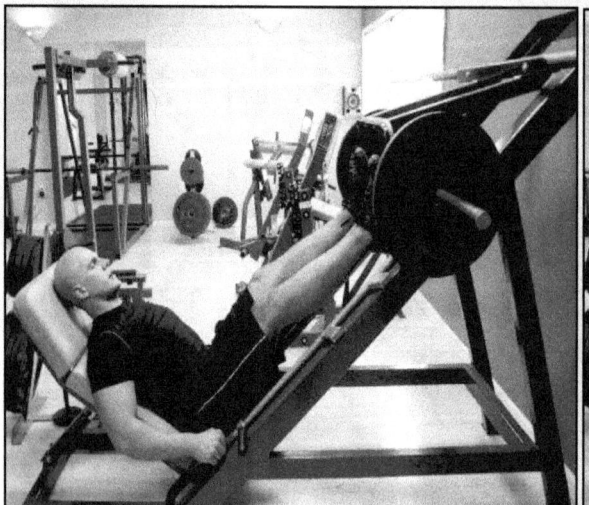
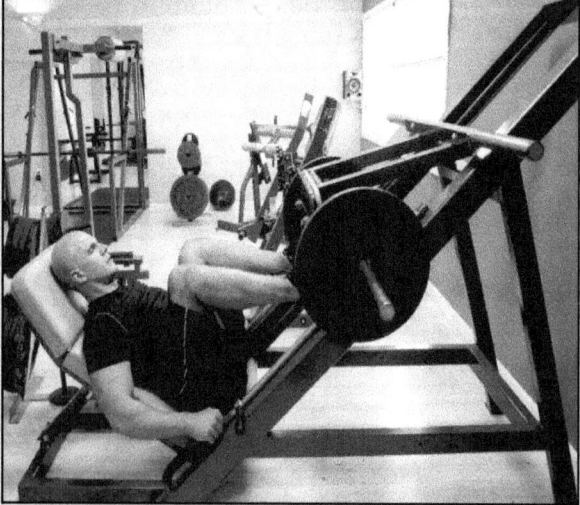

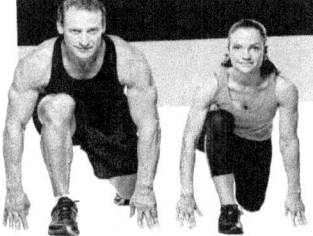

AB SESSION

HACK SQUAT MACHINE

Primary muscle(s): Quadriceps Group

Synergistic muscle(s): Gluteus Maximus, Hamstring Group

DESCRIPTION:

- Step under shoulder harnesses on a hack squat machine
- Place feet on platform, shoulder width apart
- Feet should be far enough out in front of your so you will not break knee toe line when you are in the down position
- Slowly lift weight upward and rotate safeties out of the way
- For the eccentric portion of the lift, slowly descend
- Eccentric portion of the exercise should take four seconds
- Inhale during the eccentric portion of the lift
- Continue downward until knees are parallel to the floor (90° angle)
- Maintain knee toe line
- Do not bounce at bottom of the movement (this will place unneeded stress on the patella)
- For the concentric portion of the lift, drive upward through the heels
- Concentric portion should take two seconds
- Exhale during the concentric portion of the lift
- Do not lock knees at the top of motion (this will remove the tension on the muscle and cause unneeded stress on the patella)
- Repeat for desired number of repetitions
- Once desired number of repetitions

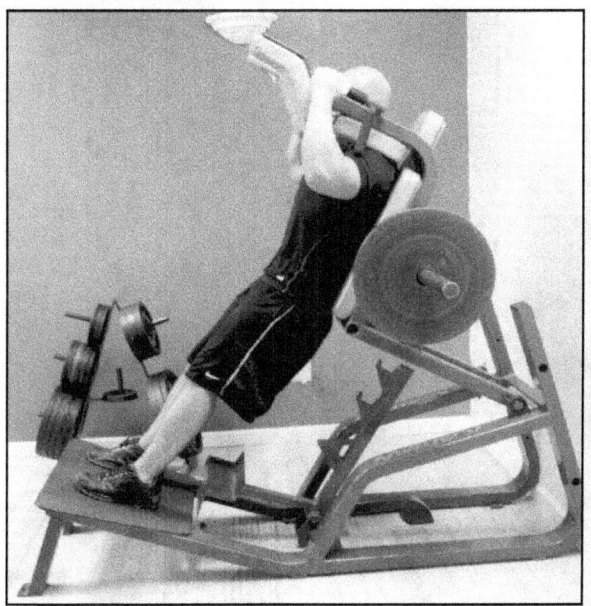
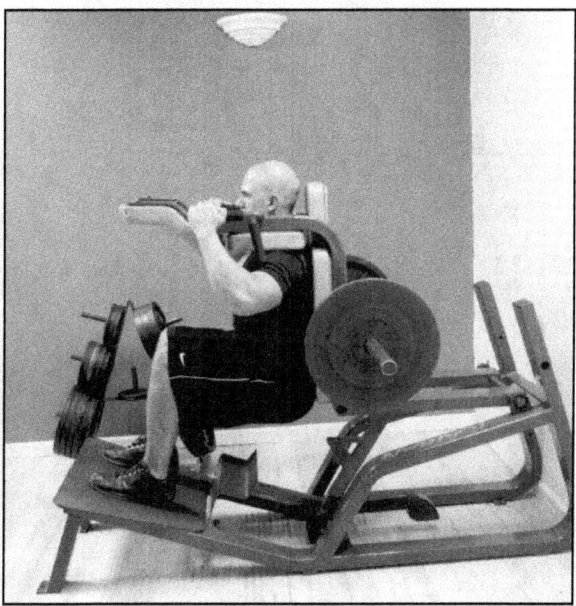

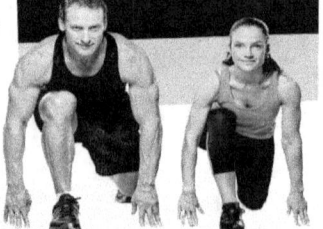

SHRUGS

BARBELL / DUMBBELLS

Primary muscle(s): Trapezius I

Synergistic muscle(s): Forearms

DESCRIPTION:

- Keep back neutral in an upright position
- Keep knees slightly bent and shoulders retracted
- Grasp bar in an overhand grip (an alternating grip – one under and one over) may also be used
- Hold bar at arm's length resting at thigh level
- Begin movement by elevating shoulders towards ears and hold (Do not roll the shoulders)
- After concentric portion slowly return to start position while obtaining a good stretch
- Repeat for desired number of repetitions

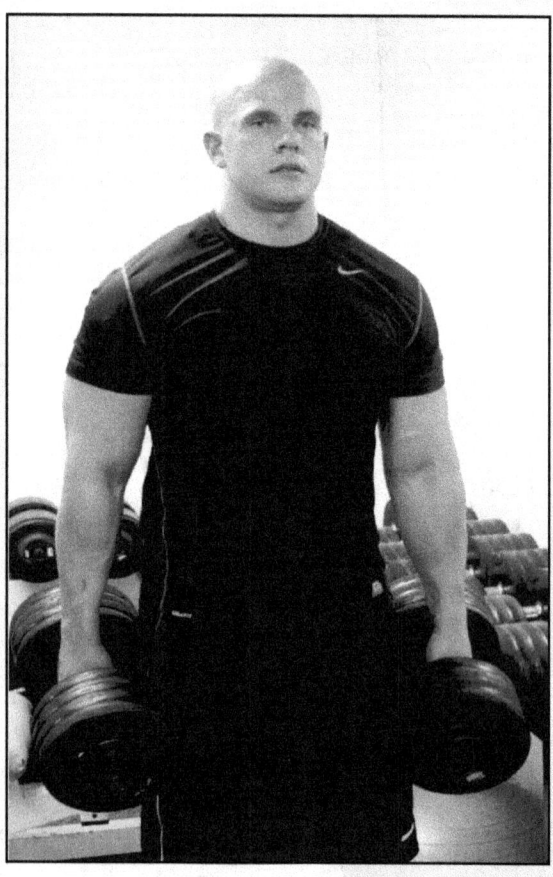
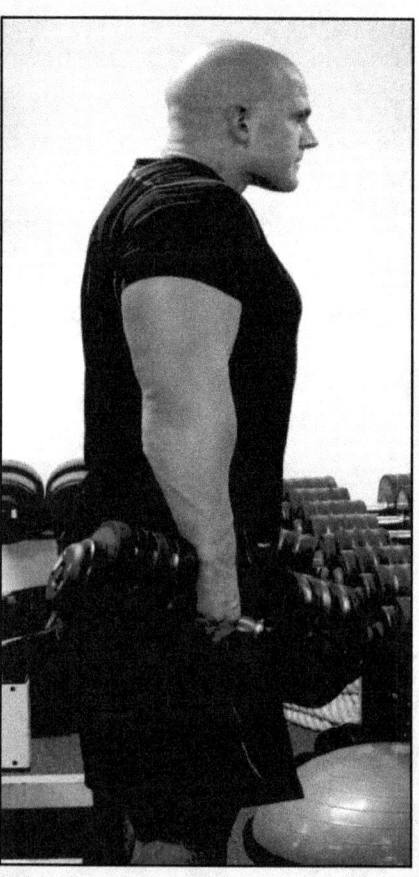

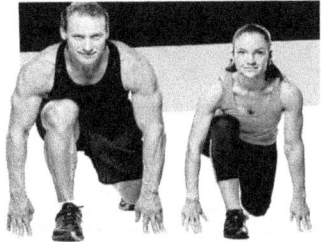

UNDERHAND CLOSE GRIP PULL UPS

PULL UP BAR

Primary muscle(s): Biceps Brachii

Synergistic muscle(s): Latissimus Dorsi

DESCRIPTION:

- Grasp chin up bar with an underhand grip closer than shoulder width apart
- Pull body up in a vertical line, until chin passes bar
- Slowly return to start position without releasing tension on muscle
- Do not return to a full hang (this will remove the tension from the biceps and place it on the shoulder joints)
- Repeat for desired number of repetitions

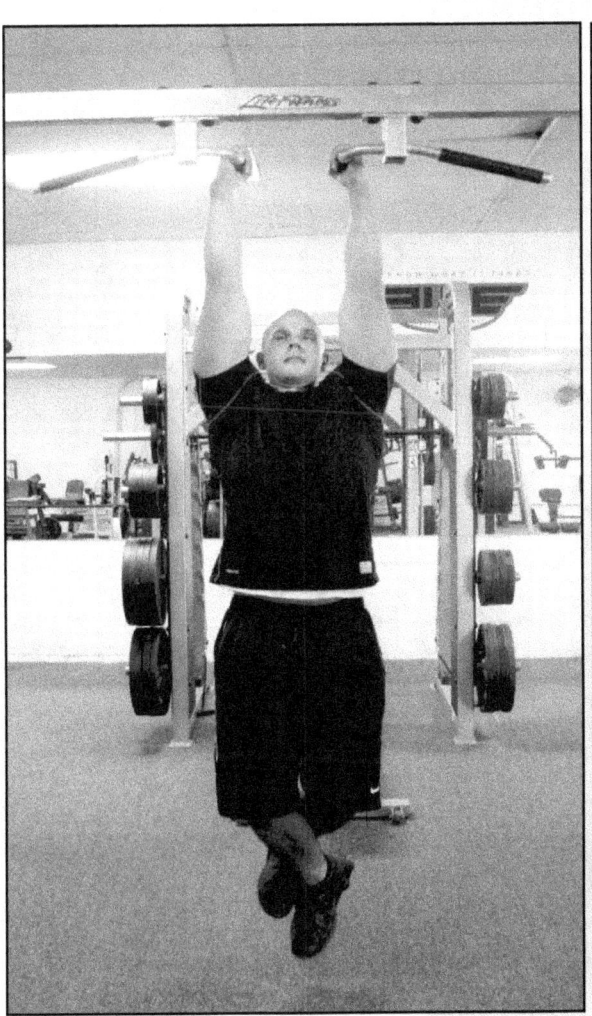
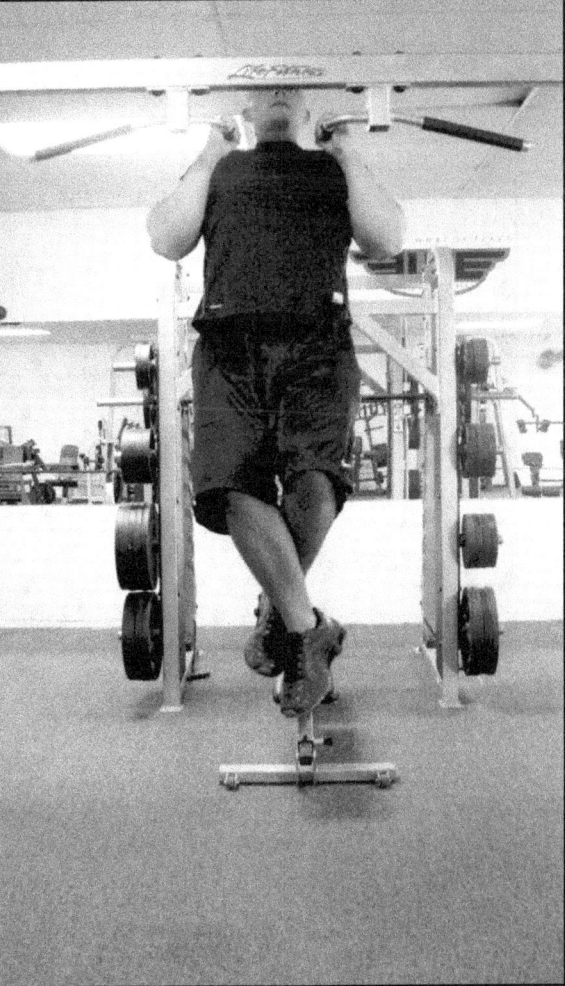

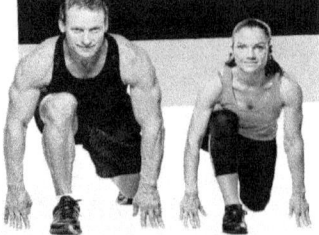

STRAIGHT BAR / EZ BAR / DUMBBELLS

Primary muscle(s): Biceps Brachii, Brachialis

Synergistic muscle(s): Forearms

DESCRIPTION:

- Grasp bar with hands supinated (underhand) slightly wider than hip width apart
- Keep knees slightly bent
- Retract scapula
- For concentric (positive) portion of the exercise, slowly raise the bar by decreasing the angle of the elbow joint
- Concentric portion should take two seconds and you should exhale
- Slowly lower bar to start position for eccentric (negative) portion of the exercise
- Eccentric portion should take four seconds to complete and you should inhale
- Repeat for desired number of repetitions

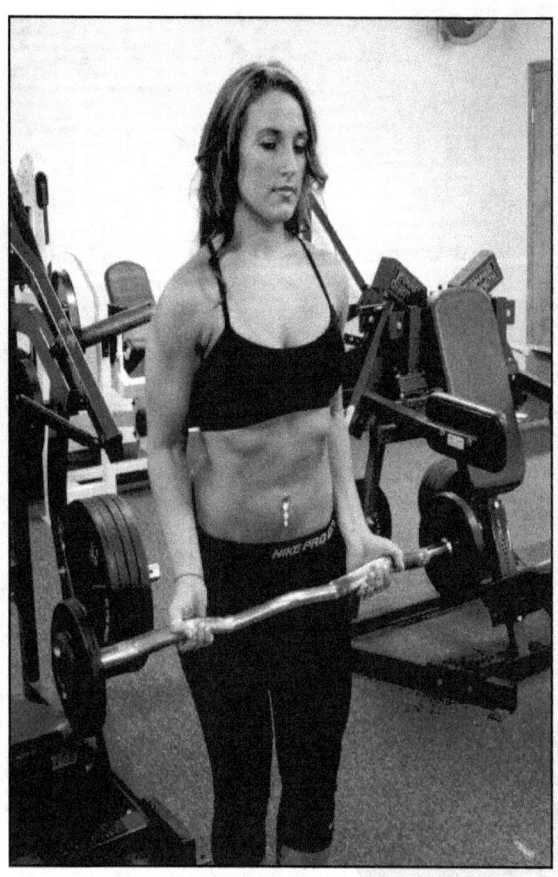
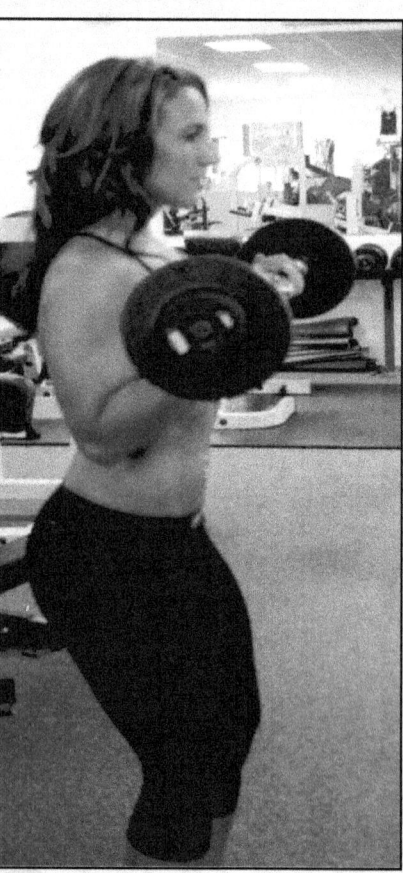

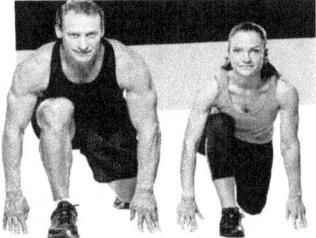

DIPS

PARALLEL BAR

Primary muscle(s): Triceps Brachii

Synergistic muscle(s): Anterior Deltoid, Pectoralis Major

DESCRIPTION:

- Begin by supporting bodyweight with arms straight between parallel bars
- For triceps- keep body in an upright position
- Bend elbows and lower body
- Lower body until elbows form a 90° angle
- Push torso back to start position by extending arms
- Do not extend arms to full lock out
- Repeat for desired number of repetitions

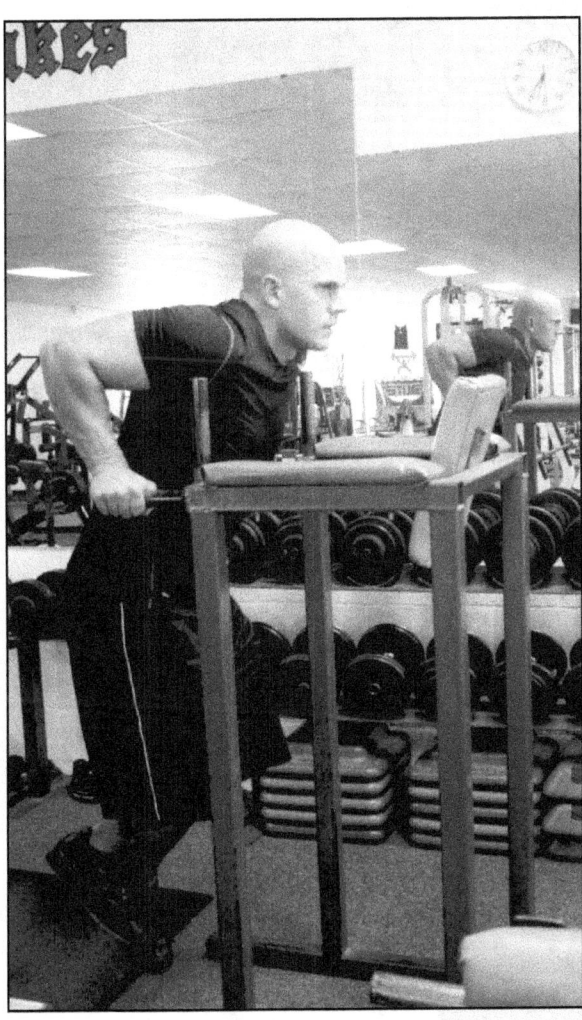
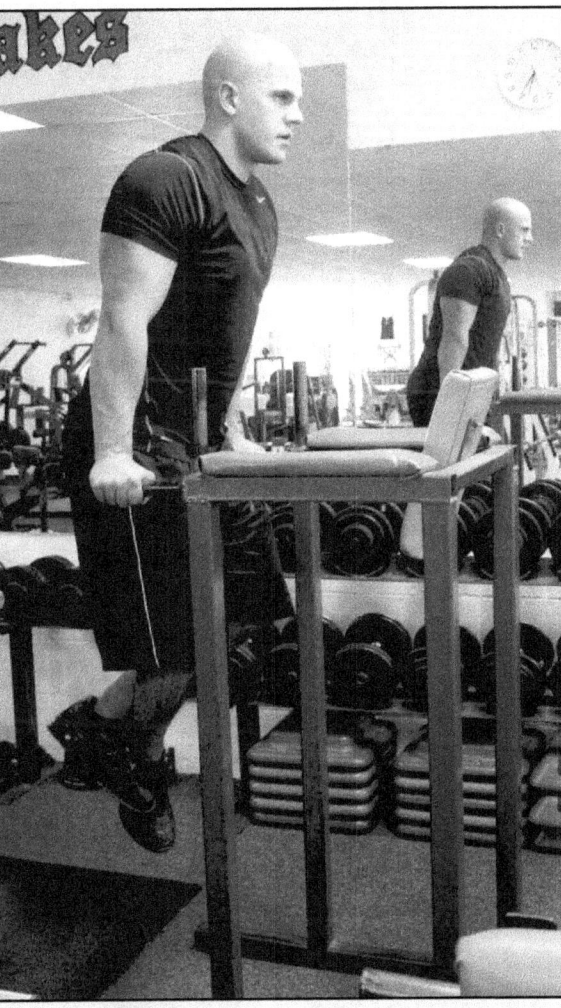

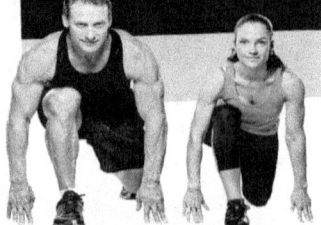

BARBELL / BENCH

Primary muscle(s): Triceps Brachii

Synergistic muscle(s): Anterior Deltoid, Pectoralis Major

DESCRIPTION:

- Position yourself on a flat bench with eyes directly under the bar
- Grasp barbell with hands slightly closer than shoulder width apart
- (If hands are too close, you will experience wrist impingement)
- Keep feet flat on floor
- Lift bar off uprights with assistance of spotter
- For eccentric portion of exercise, slowly lower bar (4 seconds) while inhaling
- Keep elbows close to body
- Drive bar back to start position (2 seconds) while

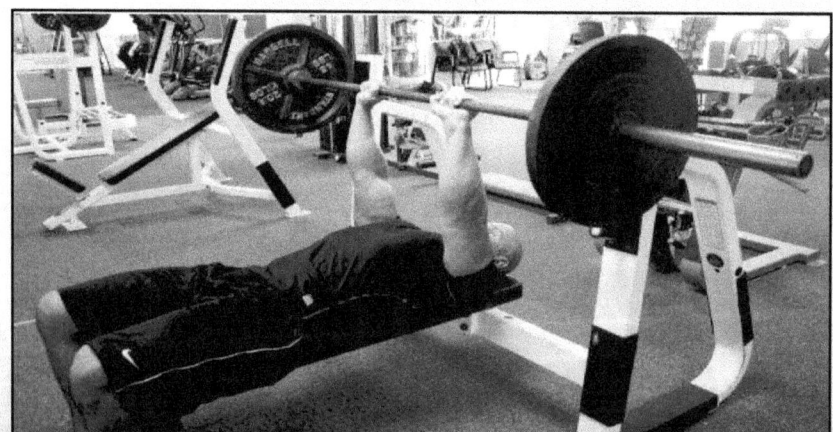

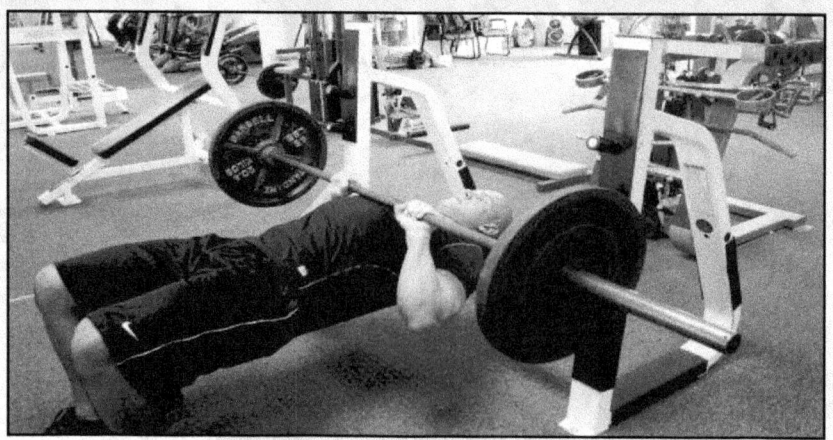

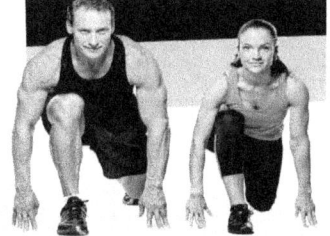

OVERHEAD DUMBBELL EXTENSIONS

DUMBBELL

Primary muscle(s): Triceps Brachii

Synergistic muscle(s):

DESCRIPTION:

- Sit on the end of a flat bench
- Grasp dumbbell with both hands with dumbbell resting on knee
- Both hands should be overlapping on one end of the dumbbell
- Rotate hands and dumbbell so it is an overhead position
- For the eccentric portion of the lift, begin by slowly lowering weight by bending the elbows
- Keep elbows pointing towards the front throughout the exercise
- Continue downward motion until elbows reach a 90° angle
- The eccentric portion of the lift should take four seconds and you should inhale
- To begin the concentric portion of the lift drive forcefully upward with arms until they return to starting position
- The concentric portion of the lift should take two seconds and you should exhale
- Do not lock arms at the top of the movement (this will place unneeded stress on the elbow joint)
- Do not bounce at bottom of the movement

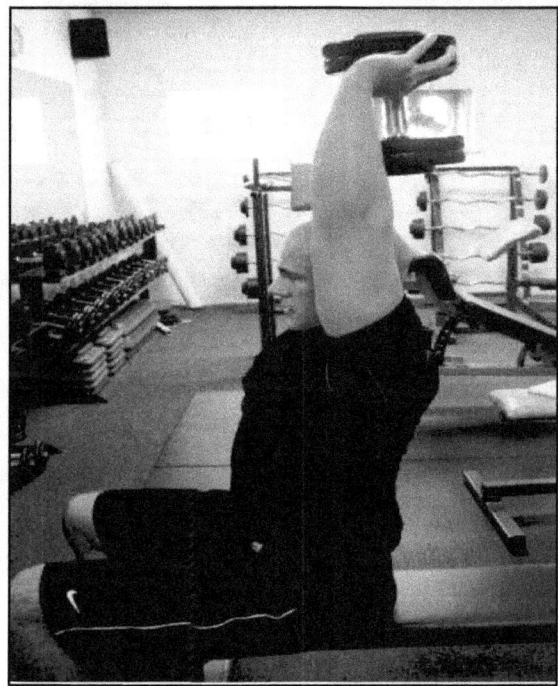
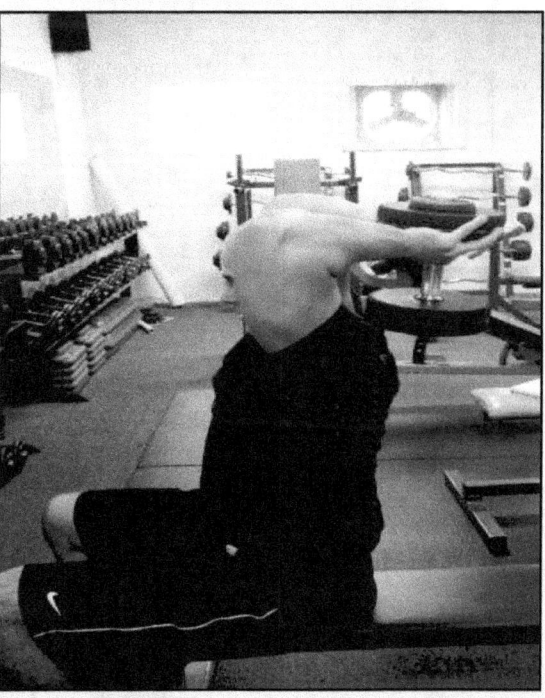

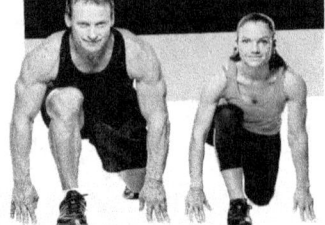

STANDING CALF RAISES

BARBELL / DUMBBELLS

Primary muscle(s): Gastrocnemius

Synergistic muscle(s): Soleus

DESCRIPTION:

- Approach bar while on squat rack uprights
- Begin by retracting scapula and placing bar on the upper Trapezius
- Keep back in a neutral arch, head facing forward during entirety of exercise
- Lift bar off of uprights and step backwards in squat rack
- Feet should be pointed forward and slightly closer than hip width apart
- Begin concentric portion by lifting heel off of the ground
- Concentric portion should take two seconds
- Exhale during concentric portion
- Return to start position, while getting a good stretch in calf
- Eccentric portion should take four seconds
- Inhale during the eccentric portion of lift
- Do not bounce at bottom of the exercise
- Complete for desired number of repetitions
- Once desired number of repetitions are completed, return bar to squat rack uprights

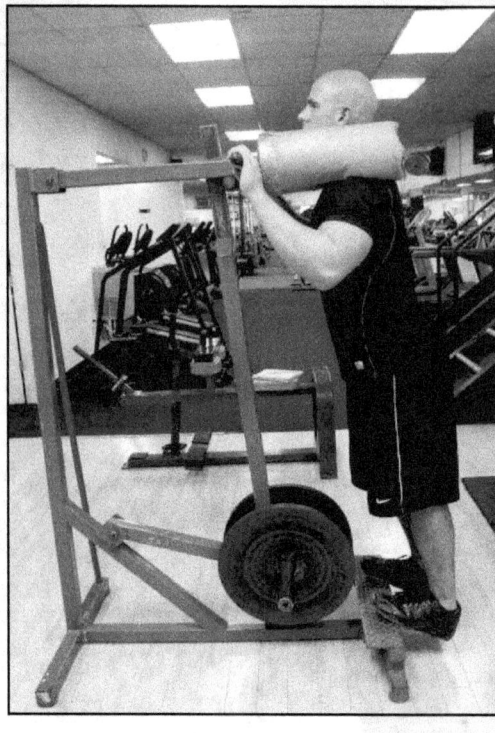
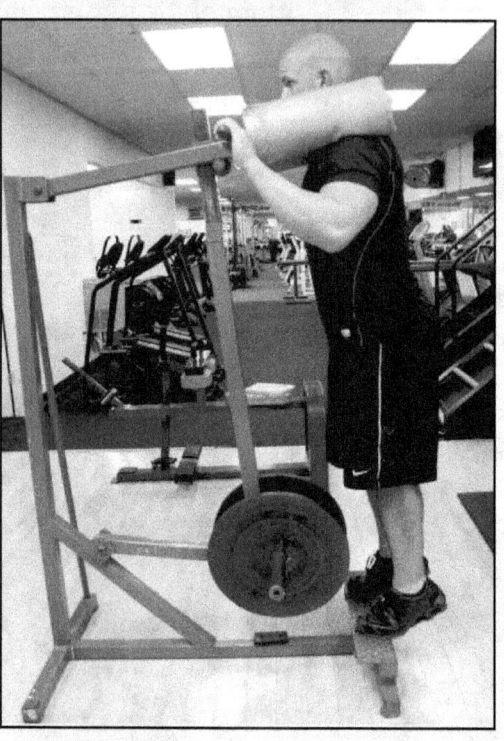

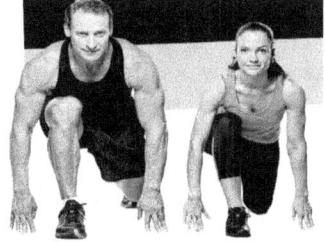

SEATED CALF RAISES

SEATED CALF MACHINE

Primary muscle(s): Soleus

Synergistic muscle(s): Gastrocnemius

DESCRIPTION:

- Sit on calf raise machine with pad secured across legs, knees bent and feet planted firmly on the foot rest
- This exercise can also be performed by sitting on the end of a flat bench and placing dumbbells or a barbell across legs
- For concentric portion of the exercise raise heels off of the foot rest (or floor if on a flat bench)
- Concentric portion of lift should take two seconds
- Exhale during concentric portion
- For eccentric portion of the lift slowly descend back to starting position while obtaining a good stretch throughout the calf
- Do not bounce at bottom of the exercise
- Once completing desired number of repetitions return weight to start position and return safety on machine

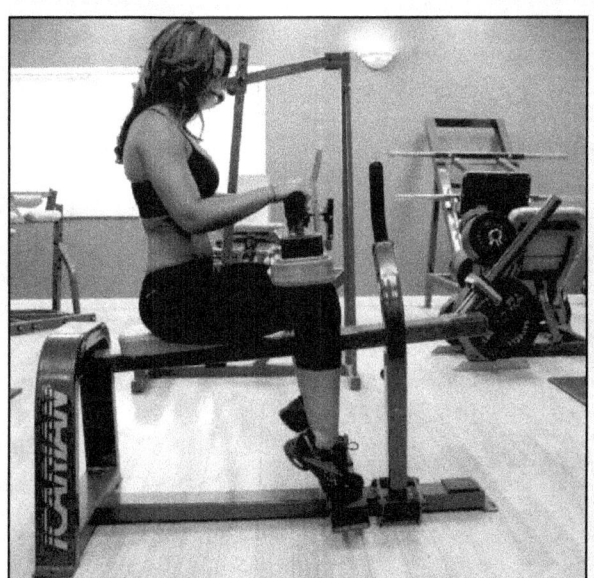
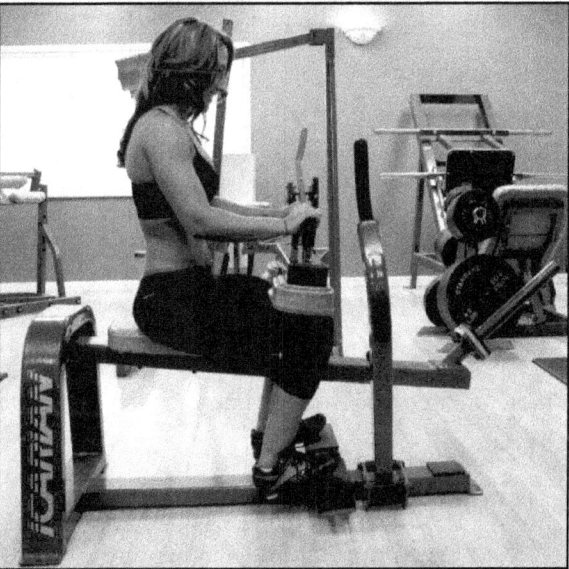

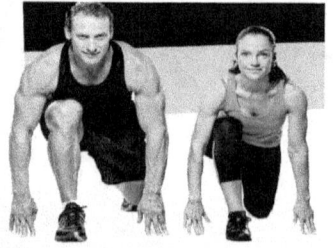

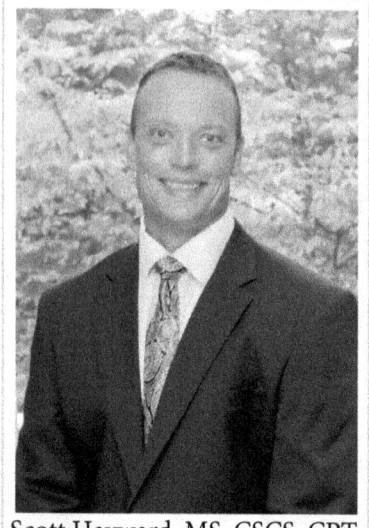

Scott Hayward, MS, CSCS, CPT

Referred to as one of the country's premier personal trainers, body transformation, and fat loss experts, Scott Hayward truly changes bodies and changes lives. As an author, lecturer, trainer, and educator, he is sought out by those looking to transform their bodies and ultimately transform their lives.

Scott, who holds numerous degrees and certifications, is the author of; ⊠Absession⊠ America⊠ Guide to Ultimate 6 Pack Abs,⊠as well as numerous articles onAnatomy, Physiology, Energy Metabolism, and Exercise Science. His seminars, lectures and workshops on on fat loss, weight loss, and body transformation techniques have transformed thousands of lives.

Scott is the consulting exercise physiologist for a fitness product development company, which has several exciting pieces of fitness equipment slated for release in the near future.

Scott owned and operated an 8,000 square foot Personal Training Facility. He was the fitness director for a 3,000 member health and fitness facility, participated in and coached college athletics and was an adjunct professor for several nationally accredited personal training certifications.

Scott is married to Jennifer Lynn Hayward and they reside in the Philadelphia region with their Siberian Husky named Zoey. Together they have formed Fit for Faith Ministries. Fit for Faith Ministries is a Christian Fitness Ministry which is dedicated to educating, inspiring and empowering people to become better stewards of the body God has given them. Fit for Faith Ministry conducts fat loss seminars and body transformation programs for churches throughout the region.

Check out Fit for Faith on the web at www.fitforfaithministries.com

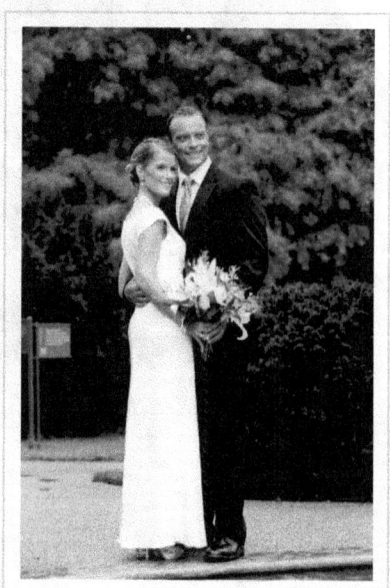